HEALTHY SEXUALITY: 3 BOOKS in 1:

INTIMACY AND DESIRE + MINDFULNESS SEX + SEXUAL INTIMACY a complete guide to reach sexual health in the couple. Positions, tantric sex and kama sutra tips.

DONNA DARE

© **Copyright 2019 - All rights reserved.**

The content contained within this book may not be reproduced, duplicated or transmitted without direct written permission from the author or the publisher.

Under no circumstances will any blame or legal responsibility be held against the publisher, or author, for any damages, reparation, or monetary loss due to the information contained within this book. Either directly or indirectly.

Legal Notice:

This book is copyright protected. This book is only for personal use. You cannot amend, distribute, sell, use, quote or paraphrase any part, or the content within this book, without the consent of the author or publisher.

Disclaimer Notice:

Please note the information contained within this document is for educational and entertainment purposes only. All effort has been executed to present accurate, up to date, and reliable, complete information. No warranties of any kind are declared or implied. Readers acknowledge that the author is not engaging in the rendering of legal, financial, medical or professional advice. The content within this book has been derived from various sources. Please consult a licensed professional before attempting any techniques outlined in this book.

By reading this document, the reader agrees that under no circumstances is the author responsible for any losses, direct or indirect, which are incurred as a result of the use of information contained within this document, including, but not limited to, — errors, omissions, or inaccuracies.

Table of Contents

INTIMACY AND DESIRE

Description 13

Introduction 17

Chapter 1 Different Types of Intimacy 25

Chapter 2 Intimacy and Sex in a Marriage .. 27

Chapter 3 How to Revive Intimacy 36

    Prioritize Your Relationship 36

    Flirt With Each Other 37

    Create a Habit 38

    Getting In the Mood 38

    Date Nights 39

    Make Them Feel Special 39

    Terms of Endearment 40

    Don't Let Yourself Go 40

    Don't Take Arguments to Bed 41

    Increase Your Physical Contact 42

Chapter 4 Creating Emotional Intimacy with Your Man 43

Chapter 5 Spice Things Up In the Sack 48

Chapter 6 Communication Practices 56

Chapter 7 Forgetting About Past Ghosts 76

Chapter 8 Loving Words Heal Relationships 90
   How to Express Love Words 94
   Using Words of Love to Inspire the Relationship - 3 Tips for Men to Learn 97

Chapter 9 What Women Want; What Men Want 100

Chapter 10 Tips to Have More Intimacy in Every Situation 106

Chapter 11 Restoring Intimacy in Your Marriage 114

Chapter 12 Tantric Sex For Marriage 120
   The Yin and the Yang: Which is male and which is female? 121
      Shiva and Shakti 122
      Understanding the opposites 123
      My partner is my beloved 124
      The Desire Spectrum 124
      You feel empowered to say what you want! 125

Chapter 13 Teachings of tantric sex 126
   Breathe 126
   Relax 129
   Sounds can help! 130
   Eye contact is essential 133
   Pay attention 135
   Always be present 136

Chapter 14 Understand the Challenges Created by Social Messages 138
- Challenges for Women 138
  - Distractibility During Sex 138
  - Loss of Sexual Interest as a Mom 139
  - Low Sexual Desire 139
- Challenges for Men 140
  - Midlife Crisis 140
  - Sexual Dysfunction 141
- Challenges for Couples 142
  - Sexless Relationship/Marriage 142
  - Emotional Distance 143
- One Couple's Plight Through the Lens of Social Messages 144

Chapter 15 Romance After The Kids 147
- Update Each Other Every Week 148
- Sharing the Parenting 149
- Finding Time for Intimacy 149
- Get Yourselves a Babysitter 151
- Pay More Attention To Your Spouse 152
- Appreciation, Admiration and Affection 153

Chapter 16 Improving Intimacy 155

Chapter 17 More Intimacy in 7 Days 163

Conclusion 176

MINDFULNESS SEX

Description 181
Introduction 184
Chapter 1 The Psychology of Sex 189
    Climate of Intimacy 191
    The Female Sexual Map.....................................193
    The Female as Identity 194
    The Clitoris..196
Chapter 2 Sex and Spirituality......................... 198
Chapter 3 Prepare Mind and Body for Sex 205
    Peace and privacy 205
    Feather the nest...207
    It's up to you to lubricate or not 208
    Bath or shower 208
Chapter 4 Keep Your Enemy Closer 210
Chapter 5 Reconnect With Your Partner 230
Chapter 6 Breathing and Diaphragmatic Breathing 243
    Breathing..244
        Re-birthing breathing 247
Chapter 7 Setting the Mood 251
    Peace and privacy 251
    Feather the nest...253
    It's up to you to lubricate or not 254
    Bath or shower 254

Chapter 8 Spin Your Chakras and Breathe To Ecstasy **256**

Chapter 9 Sexual Domination and Submission . 259

Chapter 10 Reel Life to Real Life **273**

Chapter 11 Personal Lubricants **280**

   Slippin' and a slidin' – the lubrication basics......... 281

      Water-based 282

      Silicon-based 283

      Hybrids 283

      Oil-based 284

   Where to buy it 286

Chapter 12 So you want to be a Superhero? 288

Chapter 13 Develop Sexual Intuition **295**

Chapter 14 Sexual Massages **302**

   Types of massage to try on your partner 306

      Female genital massage 306

      Male genital massage 307

      Sensual or erotic massages 308

      Body to body massage 309

Chapter 15 Mindful Oral Sex **311**

Chapter 16 Alternative Sexual Experiences **323**

Chapter 17 Would You Ever? **337**

   Role play 338

   Bondage 341

   Spanking 342

Chapter 18 Conclusion **344**

SEXUAL INTIMACY

Description **351**
Introduction **354**
   Learning to Touch *356*
   The Active Role and the Liability *357*
   Awakening the Sensations *359*
   Be Acierated from Front and Backs *360*
Chapter 1 How Communicate with Your Partner **363**
Chapter 2 Developing Your Sexual Relationship with Your Partner **366**
Chapter 3 Clearing the Decks for Sex **380**
   Tempus fugit (time flies) *381*
   Making time your bitch *383*
   Back to that "roommate" thing *386*
Chapter 4 Explore Him/Her Body **388**
   The Female Body *388*
   The Male Body *404*
Chapter 5 How to Give an Erotic Massage to Help Increase Intimacy **412**
Chapter 6 Unlocking Intimate Capacity Through Synergy **421**
Chapter 7 Spicy And Dirty Talk **439**
Chapter 8 Masturbation **449**

How to Enjoy it to the Maximum 450

In Solitude 451

In Couple 452

Chapter 9 Orgasms **455**

Chapter 10 Sex Toys: What Choose For Him And For Her **470**

Chapter 11 Using Props During Sex **482**

Chapter 12 Sexual And Aphrodisiac Food .. **489**

Chapter 13 The Intricacies of Pleasure and Orgasms **497**

Chapter 14 The Most Intimate Positions For Couple **507**

Conclusion **531**

INTIMACY AND DESIRE

How to stimulate a relationship discovering what she/he really wants into the bed. A journey into sexual fantasies in marriage and couples to have good sex and sexual health.

DONNA DARE

Description

Sexual connection and satisfaction is a key factor to a more fulfilling relationship. Many couples experience a decline of sexual desire and frequency of intercourse over the course of a long-term relationship, but studies have shown that couples who work to keep the passion alive are often happier. By viewing sex as part of the glue that binds you a greater intimacy can be achieved and a closeness that will satisfy your needs can be achieved.

Here we will examine a few key tips to keep your sex life interesting and are facts that all happy couples know are unquestionably true about having a great sex life!

Maybe you are one of those rare couples that have incredible amounts of fantastic sex even years into your relationship, and if you are, well done you, maybe you should write a book and tell everyone your secret!! If not, then read on! It is a true fact that in general the longer a couple has been together the less sex they will be having. Now that is not altogether a bad thing as long as you realize that good sex is important and as long as you are aware of the little things you do that drive your partner crazy with lust and you are still doing them. Maybe think about trying a few new moves, be creative! Providing you have a relationship that allows you to be truthful with each other the skies the limit!

Remembering that as you age and your body changes that you will both need more time to become aroused and climax. Make time for sex, forget the hurried frantic sexual encounters often reminiscent of your early years. Can it really be a bad thing to take more time having intercourse? Think about it, a relaxed interruption free atmosphere, great surroundings and comfortable locations can only improve matters. In fact, by taking more time and introducing new relaxed techniques you can open up all-new experiences. Make sure you take time to show physical affection when having sex. Kissing for long periods of time can lead to heightened emotions and a greater feeling of sharing a physical bond. It is important to feel connected during this most intimate of acts and by avoiding distractions and committing yourself fully this can be achieved.

Honesty plays a huge part in maintaining a healthy sex life. You may feel that by faking an orgasm you are shielding your partner's feelings but you are creating a dangerous precedent. By starting an honest and meaningful conversation about your physical needs, your expectations and dislikes you can open up the door to a deeply satisfying experience for both of you. Avoid criticism and learn how to suggest positive actions rather than focusing on negative issues. Confide in your partner any changes you would like to try, research new positions and sex aids that you would both be comfortable with! Research can be fun, giggling over the wild and wacky range of toys that are out there and can be found on the internet can bring you closer together. Whilst many couples find it hard to talk about sex good communication is essential to healthy relationships.

This guide will focus on the following:

- Different types of intimacy
- Intimacy and sex in a marriage
- How to revive intimacy

- Creating emotional intimacy with your man
- Spice things up in the sack
- Communication practices
- Things to do as a couple
- Loving words heal relationships
- What women want; what men want
- Tips to have more intimacy in every situation
- Restoring intimacy in your marriage
- Tantric sex for marriage
- Teachings of tantric sex
- Understand the challenges created by social messages
- Romance after the kids
- Improving intimacy
- More intimacy in 7 days... AND MORE!!!

Introduction

Experimentation is essential to maintain healthy interest. Compare your love life to your daily diet, for instance, how would you feel if you were served the same meal, at the same time and on the same plate day after day? Bored, right? So, change things up a bit! Sexual positions are a start, often we rely on tried and trusted sexual positions and that is great for the majority of the time but every now and again explore some new moves! As long as you are aware of your own and your partners' limitations physically you can find new ways to increase stimulation. By choosing new positions you can also overcome problems caused by physical limitations.

Understand the different actions that can be classed as foreplay. Often mundane tasks can become the main activity of a normal day, realizing the potential of these everyday activities can be eye-opening. For instance, if your partner decides to take on one of your least favorite household tasks and maybe vacuums the whole house because he knows you hate doing it, then they are trying to make you happy and that can be one of the sexiest things ever!! Foreplay is often overlooked by people in a long-term relationship and this can lead to resentment and disappointment that will eventually lead to problems both in the bedroom and outside.

Foreplay can often start with the basic act of preparing for intimacy. By dressing sexily, maybe lingerie and a slinky nightie, fixing your hair and adding a bit of make-up can all lead to heightened confidence. Confidence is a major boost to your levels of sexiness and can lead to increased ability to take it that bit further when switching things up!

Maybe the man is the traditional leader in the bedroom, imagine how fun it would be to swap those roles over. Always maintaining awareness of the other partner's feelings, change the roles in the boudoir, there is always the potential for surprise when it comes to making out!

Masturbation is often regarded as a solo activity but can be a fantastic foreplay tool. Showing your partner that you are in control of your own sexuality can be a major turn on. Invite them to join in and you can quite often create a mutual sense of satisfaction. Take it slow and steady and you will find that exploring your partner's methods of masturbation and self-pleasuring can give you interesting ideas when it is your turn to give them pleasure! Think of it as a pleasurable insight into what floats your partner's boat!

Exercise is a great way to improve sexual fitness. Often over time our bodies can become less taut and both sexes can benefit from some simple pelvic floor muscle exercises. One simple method that can be used by both men and women is to contract your bladder as if trying to prevent urination. Do this contraction 5 to 10 times a go and at half a dozen different times of the day. By doing so you are exercising the muscles that contract during orgasm. By flexing and toning these muscles you augment the sensations and make it easier to achieve a satisfying orgasm.

These exercises also tighten the vaginal muscles and increase the flow of blood to the pelvic area meaning that both partners will enjoy a more intense and pleasurable experience during sex.

Whilst they were originally developed to aid relief for people who had given birth or had been involved in accidents it is widely believed that by practicing these simple exercises you can improve not only your sex life but the general control over bladder and bowel. The pelvic floor is also known as your pelvic diaphragm and by increasing the amount of time tightening up these muscles a marked difference in all areas associated with the area should be evident. It is worth pointing out that whilst the exercises replicate the action of stopping urine mid-flow it is actually very dangerous to do so whilst urinating.

A great way to perk up your libido is by removing household objects from your bedroom. It can be distracting to find yourself looking at the picture of granddad on the nightstand, work clothes scattered about the room can just make you think about work-related stuff. Make your bedroom a retreat, use soft colors and materials, think sexy boudoir rather than working bedroom and your mind, and body will respond to these extra stimuli.

Ditch the TV! In the bedroom especially how many of us have fallen asleep to the dulcet tones of some late-night presenter when really, we would love to be falling asleep exhausted by our love lives? Move the goggle box into the den and take time out to talk to each other before sleep. The good old make-out session can soon be replacing mind-numbing TV watching. If that is working for you why not try the same trick in the lounge? If you are not brave enough to ditch it completely the at least set a schedule to turn it off on certain nights.

Don't ignore problems. Whilst erectile dysfunction is a common sexual problem and affects a number of men much less is known about women's problems and how to treat them. Later in life, many women experience vaginal dryness and pain due to lack of lubrication. If lubrication is needed there are many forms of artificial alternatives to choose from. Good old KY jelly can make intercourse a pleasure again. Why not try to make an application a form of foreplay? Often a woman can be too embarrassed to address this condition as it often occurs at the same time as menopause and can lead to feelings of uselessness and somehow feeling less womanly.

A thoughtful and loving partner will be able to take a potentially distressing situation and use it to restore a feeling of sexiness in his partner. Make sure you lubricate slowly and sensually and you will both derive pleasure from the sensations you will arouse. Done correctly this will lead to pain-free and very slippery sex, now who doesn't want that??

The best sex is achieved by taking on board your partner's feelings, fears and hopes and by being the best that you can be you will work together and achieve the ultimate goal, love intimacy and satisfaction.

Recapitulating, intimacy issues are not just intimacy issues. As the sexual activity is a basic instance for pleasure-seeking, whatever happens in it works as a symptom of something else, more general and profound, related to the way we pursue what we want in life. One does not fail at sex, one *also* fails at sex. Why also there? Because it works as the ultimate and key surface where our unconscious self can express itself. Quite often, we do not realize (or deny) what we are passing through until we feel some discomfort or frustration in our sexual life that makes us ask ourselves about it.

In other words, we cannot lie to ourselves in bed as we may do it in other aspects of our lives. We may lie to our partner, but definitely not to ourselves. As long as sex and intimacy are such particular experiences for every person and couple, there is no universal rule to identify if you are failing at it or not. So, the best way to know it is to determine it yourself. Additionally, 'failing' is not a good word to describe intimacy issues. There is nothing a goal to reach but to find what gives you and your partner pleasure.

Just be extremely honest with you: Do you enjoy your sexual life? Do you feel confident with your partner? Do you have as much sex as you want? Do you reach orgasms with your partner? Do you feel that you would prefer to be with someone else? Do you feel your sexual activity is satisfactory to yourself? Do you want to do something you have never done before but you are not sure about how your partner will react?

Ask yourself these questions and others. Try to find what really separates you from the place you would want to be. As 'failing' is an inaccurate word to talk about sex and intimacy, the same happens with the idea of 'fault'.

Sexuality is something shared, and (in principle) develops in the context of a couple. Nothing means anything without its context, and what could be good for a couple will not for another one. In the same sense, things only happen in their specific coordinates, and would not be possible in other scenarios. What we mean is that if something happens in the sexual life of a couple it will be both people's business. The responsibility is shared as well. Even if whatever happens seems to affect just one person, both should take it as a serious issue that needs to be discussed.

Chapter 1 Different Types of Intimacy

You might be surprised, but there are different types of intimacy in relationships. The two primary types of intimacy are physical and emotional. Because of this, different partners are likely to see different types of intimacy as more important. You and your partner might have two different ideas of what intimacy should look like in your relationship, so it is important that you learn to communicate with these types of things.

Physical intimacy is an intimacy that is shown through physical touch. People who are more interested in physical intimacy tend to feel more connected to their partner through touch. The touch can be non-sexual such as hand-holding, a hand on the shoulder, hugging, and even sitting next to each other with body parts touching. Or, it can be sexual. When you want to turn someone on who is more interested in physical intimacy, you need to use this to your advantage. Use sensual touching of various areas of the body as an opportunity to turn them on.

Emotional intimacy is an intimacy that is given and received through feelings. People who are more interested in emotional intimacy are turned on through words and other things that evoke emotions. They may be more likely to respond to surprises, storytelling, gifts, and more.

Most relationships rely on both types of intimacy, though the balance will be unique to each individual relationship. Finding the perfect balance will require communication and practice as you both learn how to physically and emotionally communicate with each other in a way that nurtures your relationship.

Chapter 2 Intimacy and Sex in a Marriage

Sex in marriage enhances the bond between two partners. It should form part of how two partners interact and express their love for each other. The common belief is that humans might find it hard to mate for life. That is not the case; there are innovative ways to make sex interesting so that partners enjoy each other for life. Some creativity reignites the spark in bed leaving your partner yearning for you every time. Choose to believe that it is not difficult to make sex seem new every time. The right attitude makes sex as interesting as if was the first time.

Sex is as much mental as it is physical. Partners should share a deep connection so that they are always in sync in any activity they carry out together. Sex is one element that requires this sort of connection for it to be totally fulfilling. A sexless marriage is a major problem in many marriages. One spouse may be desperately yearning for touch and physical closeness and when these needs are ignored a major disconnect happens. The spouse may feel unwanted, unappreciated and the couple even stops spending time together. Eye contact lessens and the bond between them weakens and puts the marriage in a risky position. This chapter will focus on the frequently asked questions about sex in marriage and how to deal with them.

The most common question asked about sex is whether it is possible to keep sex interesting after being with your partner for such a long time. Well, it is very possible. There are different ways to ensure that sex remains part of a married couple's life that they always look forward to. It takes a little effort but it is worthwhile since you are with your partner for a lifetime. All it takes is a little cuddling, some new sex positions, love notes, and other simple techniques.

Seduction in marriage can still remain as tantalizing as ever. Sure, it may change with time but it can still be erotic. Partners may explore their sexuality by wearing sexy outfits for each other; especially for women. Even though people have been together for a long time, they should not give up on pleasing their partners. Sexual banter works wonders to rekindle those sexual desires. A woman can decide to visit a sex shop and choose from a wide variety of items they are comfortable with like crotch-less panties, lingerie and feminine wear that is revealing and provokes sexual tension in men. Men are visual creatures and seducing a man may need something like this. Such aspects make sex life wild and more interesting. Partners should look into ways of bringing new experiences into the sex life.

The difficulty with seduction is when two partners have different fetishes. Most couples complain of their partners taking fetishes too far. Some partners hurt each other to derive satisfaction. It has taken a toll on a lot of couples. The reasonable thing to do is to discuss with their partners and even consider the possibility of seeing a therapist. A woman once complained of her sex life with her husband deteriorating over the course of the marriage. It reached a point where the husband would slap her painfully on the face. Such a case demonstrates the way fetishes can be taken too far. Another case is where a man complained of the wife insisting on giving him a prostate massage. The man was very adamant and it formed a basis for argument and disagreement. Seduction and sex should be done under mutual consent, willingness and trust. It does not have to make your partner feel uncomfortable.

The other most commonly asked question about sex in marriage is about erectile dysfunction. Such an issue weighs down sexual energy in a marriage. Erectile dysfunction is a major cause of unhappiness in so many marriages. Sometimes, a woman may feel unattractive and the man may feel a lot of pressure by not being able to satisfy his wife. If the man is not suffering from any medical condition that predisposes them to erectile dysfunction, most of the times it is usually psychological. Medical conditions that predispose one to erectile dysfunction include diabetes. Other habits also cause erectile dysfunction like smoking and inactivity. Men should watch their cholesterol levels.

Erectile dysfunction caused by anxiety can be addressed by communication. The man has to feel the burden of pressure lifted off his chest. A therapist could help in opening up the bottled up feelings so that the man feels comfortable discussing it. Performance anxiety is a major cause of erectile dysfunction. Men with erectile dysfunction often ignore their wives and don't want to have sex which may aggravate tension in the marriage. Marriage counselors also handle a lot of cases like this. For a marriage to move on from this, communication between the partners has to be open and always at its best. Though it may take time, most couples regain their sexual vigor when psychological issues are out of the way. At a later age, women suffer reduced vaginal lubrication and reduced muscle spasms during an orgasm. Such physical hindrances can be addressed by using lubricants and estrogen replacement therapy.

Communication also helps when sex drives differ. In some marriages, sex drive is at different levels where partners are out of sync and may feel disconnected. The only way to solve this is to communicate and talk about their expectations and reason that could be affecting their libido. Sometimes, it could be work-related, family-related or so on. Couples often forget to be thankful for their strong points and choose to focus on how little sex they have in a month rather than just speaking their minds out. Talking about such issues brings synchrony where it could be lacking. As long as the minds are in sync, there will be a middle ground that will be found in sexual matters. As mentioned, even erectile dysfunction can be addressed by simply communicating.

The other commonly asked question about sex is whether exercise helps. Exercise is a major booster of a married couple's sex life. Exercise improves the overall fitness of the body and makes you more attractive. It also improves one confidence which is a major component to pleasing your partner in bed. Through exercise, people acquire endurance and energy to have sex. It sends a variety of 'feel-good hormones' throughout the body which implies a positive effect even to their partners. The effort put into exercise also makes your partner desire you more and appreciate your dedication to staying attractive for them.

Concern about the monotony of sex arises in most couples who have been married for a long time. Sex does not have to be monotonous in marriage. There are a lot of sex advice books both online and in book stores. It helps to read such books some times. Setting the mood for sex is also one way to break the monotony. Setting the mood should be done way in advance before having sex. It can be done by sending texts throughout the day to each other or starting foreplay before you even get into bed and so on. Ignoring your spouse throughout the day is one way to kill the mood. Communication helps keep the flame alive and yields positive lovemaking at the end of the day.

Often, couples compare their sex lives with others. The issue of sex should be private and should not be compared. Couples often forget that sex cannot be perfect every time as portrayed in movies or as friends would put it. Sometimes, it has its imperfection which is quite normal. To maintain the eagerness between each other, couples can try to abstain and build up desire for each other. It is the little things that make sex more interesting. Trying to look for perfect sex is futile and partners have to understand each other every time. For example, an issue that affects men psychologically is penis size. Many men sometimes feel inadequate about the size of their penis. Truthfully, it's all in the mind. When men worry too much about their penis size it can even likely cause erectile dysfunction. It is not just about the size of the penis but it's much deeper. The synchrony has to be there. Orgasms are achieved by your partner feeling they can trust you to sexually arouse them. Connect with your partner at an intimate level and the orgasm will come naturally. Women, for the most part, do not really place much concern on the size of the penis. Therefore, it is better to avoid placing emphasis on comparisons. Marriage is much more than that.

It is important to note that sex life changes as people age in a marriage. Surveys conducted indicate that as couples age in marriage, the average number of times they have sex a year decreases with time. The interesting fact is that it should not be interpreted as dissatisfaction. Most of the couples say that they are still satisfied and that they did not feel that the 'grass is greener on the other side'. This implies that sex life in marriage evolves for the better and couples should not try to be like they were in the past. Change is normal and should be expected as long the communication aspect of the marriage keeps getting better. Communication allows partners to discover what ignites that spark in their hearts and minds. It could be that it just needs going out on a romantic dinner or just as simple as taking a bubble bath together.

Sex also needs to have an element of unpredictability in a marriage. Romance and intimacy require breaking the habit of being too predictable. Falling into a comfort zone is often the case with couples but much more is needed if strengthening of the bond has to happen. It may help if partners to make a list of things they would like to venture into in the bedroom or elsewhere and place them in a jar. Every time they get an idea, they put it down and place it in the jar. Every week, they can dip their hands in the jar and do what the fantasy requires. This reignites the spark every time and the thought of not knowing what's next makes it even more worthwhile.

Chapter 3 How to Revive Intimacy

When one or both partners in a marriage or relationship are not happy, intimacy becomes a thing of the past. If one party isn't feeling loved, or doesn't feel as though the other finds them attractive anymore, instead of trying to improve themselves by dressing up or putting a bit more effort into their appearance, the opposite often occurs, making intimacy even less of an occurrence.

Other factors can contribute to the decrease of intimacy as well. These can include work, health, tiredness and children. To revive the intimacy in your relationship you need to put a bit of effort in, but it may not be as difficult as it seems.

Prioritize Your Relationship

With so many distractions and interferences in our day to day lives, it is easy to push aside the relationship. Often this is just because so many other things need to be done, and there doesn't always seem to be enough hours in the day. To revive the intimacy, one tip is to make your relationship a priority. Two or three times a week set aside a bit of time for you and your partner to be alone. It doesn't have to be a major event – it could just be going for a walk, having a coffee and a chat, or anything you might both enjoy. But you need to do it together with nobody else around. This will enable both partners to feel more connected to each other, and therefore increase the intimacy.

Flirt With Each Other

Remember back to when you first started dating, and how you used to flirt with each other. This shouldn't stop just because you are married – it should still be an important part of your relationship. Texts, emails or little notes to each other can be very stimulating on many levels. It will bring a smile to the recipient's face, and add a little anticipation to what may lie ahead at the end of the day. Flirting can also be successfully achieved by surprising your partner by dressing up more than usual. If they see you in your sweat pants on a daily basis, coming home to a wife dressed to the nines in a pair of heels will certainly get things going!

Create a Habit

A habit or a ritual that you do together can make each partner feel more connected to the other. For many couples, it is the simple ritual of kissing goodbye in the morning, and again when you see each other at the end of the day. But it can be any activity you wish, such as watching a regular television program together or saying I love you before you go to sleep at night. Whatever ritual you create, you need to follow it through every day.

Getting In the Mood

Sex drives can vary tremendously through different periods in our lives, and more often than not, one partner's drive will be higher than the other's. A lot of couples will just wait until they are both in the mood, but with the variance in the drives, this could go on for quite some time. So, you need to try and get yourself into the mood for sex regularly. This may mean exploring what it is that arouses you, or makes you feel sexy.

Date Nights

This is becoming more and more popular, and it's a great way to have some time alone together whilst doing something enjoyable. Think back to what you used to do before jobs, mortgages and kids came along. Go out to your favorite restaurant, or send the kids to the grandparents and have a candlelit dinner at home. Nothing provokes intimacy more than good food, soft music and candlelight. Or, if you are more of the adventurous couple, go out and do an activity you will both enjoy. Perhaps you could both go to dancing lessons once a week, or go see a movie. Just so long as you do something together once every week to keep those sparks going.

Make Them Feel Special

It's the little things in life that you can do for one another that can make your partner feel more special and loved. Think about something they really like, and surprise them with it without them having to ask for it. This could be cooking them their favorite dinner, serving breakfast in bed, or maybe getting that new book they wanted to read. If you are leaving the house before them, leave them a little note telling them to enjoy their day and that you love them. Letting your partner know you love them and doing little things for them will make them feel special and increase the intimacy between you.

Terms of Endearment

How many couples, when they first started dating, came up with pet names for each other? These terms of endearment are special and intimate, and there is no reason why they shouldn't continue throughout your marriage. It doesn't have to be some crazy little nickname like snuggle bunny; it could just be a name like dear, or darling. When you started out in your relationship, that nickname was brought about by how you felt about your partner. Continuing to use it reminds them that you still feel that way. It's also very important to tell your partner you love them regularly. We often lose sight of that, and being reminded that you are loved can be a great boost to any marriage.

Don't Let Yourself Go

This is just as important for women as it is for men. Yes, it's true that it can be difficult to maintain an ideal physical image, particularly as we age, or as life becomes busy. But, it is nice for both partners to see their significant other making a bit of effort to look good. You don't have to look like a superstar of course, but you shouldn't spend days on end in the same clothes with your hair in a mess either! More often than not, when you put a bit of effort into your appearance it can do wonders for your self-esteem, and that alone can make you more desirable to your partner.

Don't Take Arguments to Bed

The bedroom is the place in your house that should be reserved for showing affection and love to one another, so it shouldn't be tainted by ongoing disputes or arguments. Make a pact with your partner that you will always try to resolve any issues before you even enter the bedroom. Don't go to sleep angry, as you will still feel the same in the morning. Also, by carrying an argument into the bedroom, you will find you drift apart in the bed, and with no cuddling, caressing or pillow talk, this will create a divide between you and ruin the intimacy.

Increase Your Physical Contact

A little touch from your partner here or there throughout the day and evening can invoke a sense of intimacy. It could be a simple touch on the back in passing, or more involved such as a neck massage. The neck is quite a sensuous part of the body, and the massage works by relaxing the muscles and therefore relaxing the body. This relaxation technique can help get you in the mood for intimacy.

Chapter 4 Creating Emotional Intimacy with Your Man

If you want to create emotional intimacy, you need to lay the groundwork and actually see how he is *responding* to it. If you've been reading this book, you've likely figured out that creating this environment fertile to emotional intimacy is a lot of work.

But how do you know if he's responding the way you want? It can be difficult.

When you voice your emotions to your partner, how does he react?

If you are upset or angry or happy or nervous, you should put these feelings to direct words. Again, expecting him to read your mind is a one-way ticket to disaster.

However, when you voice your feelings... how does he react? Does he react with positive affirmations, or at least acknowledgment? Or does he seem disinterested? In healthy emotional relationships, partners at least acknowledge each other's feelings, even if they don't agree with them. If your man seems distant or completely uninterested in what you're feeling, that's a danger sign.

On the flip side, if you want to create an environment of emotional intimacy, you need to acknowledge when your man speaks to you about his emotions. Many men love it when their female partners act as an emotional sounding board. It makes them feel loved and appreciated.

Communicate directly with him. Again. Do not hint. If you want to spend more time with your man, do not attempt to do this by making him *jealous* by flirting with other men at the bar. This sends mixed signals and will absolutely not get you the response that you want.

If you express yourself in a clear and positive manner, you will get the results you want. Likewise, don't take his truthfulness as a personal attack. If you ask him how that dress looks on you and he doesn't like the dress... don't fly off the handle at him about it. You asked, and he responded. It doesn't mean he thinks you are unattractive. He simply didn't like the dress.

If you can engage in clear and constructive conversation and criticism of each other, it will actually deepen your intimacy because both of you know that your opinions are safe with each other.

Accept him and do not try to change him. Women are notorious for trying to mold their men into perfect relationship-material, and *this does not work*. The only person that you can change is yourself. Of course, there are some examples of this. If your man is a smoker and he decides that he wishes to quit, you can absolutely emotionally support him through being weaned off nicotine.

However, in this example, you are *helping* your man change in a way that he has decided on his own to do. If he doesn't want to quit smoking, demanding that he stop because *you* want him to is ineffective. Either accept that your man smokes cigarettes, or consider it a deal-breaker and move on.

This also goes with emotions. If you tell your man that you really, really like him and he changes the subject or looks uncomfortable or otherwise does not respond with the same amount of affection that you do... do not try to get him to "love you more."

This has to happen at its own pace. If it isn't happening, it isn't.

Likewise, if you want to create that awesome environment of intimacy, you definitely need to reciprocate his own displays of affection! If he tells you he loves you or adores you or wants you, make sure to tell him back in kind if you feel the same way!

Be open about sex. Obviously, if you want to fuck his brains out you need to be open and engaged with sex. However, it's important to figure out how both you and he react to each other in this manner. Do you feel inhibited or shy when bringing something up to him that you desire sexually? Are you hoping that sex will actually translate into him spending more time with you or giving you the affection that you crave?

Sex should be about sex alone. It is not a weapon that should be used to hurt your man, and it's not an item that should be exchanged for other commodities like love. You also should feel free to talk to your partner about your sexual desires. Of course, different people have different sexual desires - some may feel that mild bondage is extremely kinky, while others already have a dungeon set up in their basement for play.

The idea is not that you and your man can't have limits on what you will or won't do during sex, but that you are okay with talking about sex and you don't feel as though you'll be judged for bringing up things that you desire. For instance, some people couldn't imagine a sex life without anal, while others find the entire concept disgusting. For a great sex life, you need to be compatible in this manner.

Chapter 5 Spice Things Up In the Sack

It can be easy to fall into the same-old-same-old when it comes to sex with your man, and that's not good for him or you. You can ensure to keep on blowing his mind by keeping things a little more interesting. If you're not sure where to start, we can help you out with that!

Get all dressed up. Nothing like a little bit of clothing fun to make things a bit different. Lingerie is probably the most traditional thing here, but you can always make it a bit more exciting with French maid costumes or the like. Don't forget that he can always get dressed up, too! Maybe he could dress up like a sexy air conditioner repairman. (Just a suggestion.)

Don't look away. The next time you have sex with your man, try keeping your eyes open the entire time. You may not even realize it, but you very likely have a tendency to close your eyes during sex and escape off into your own little world. If you keep your eyes focused on your partner during sex, you may very well be surprised at how intimate the moment can become. (Hey, spicing it up isn't *just* about getting wilder than normal! Getting more emotionally intimate than normal can be extremely powerful!)

Get down with the Kama Sutra. There's a reason why this book has been around for centuries, and it's largely because it has a bunch of amazing sex moves in it. Some of the moves in the Kama Sutra are... astoundingly complex and probably shouldn't be attempted unless you are a gymnast, but there are some that are considerably more doable in nature.

For instance, consider trying **making a fire**, where you rub your husband's erect penis like you're trying to start a fire with a stick. You may also try **spiraling the stalk**, which is where you put one hand on top of another and twist them in opposite directions. **The thousand yonis** is a move where you put one hand on the top of his penis and stroke down, followed immediately by the other hand. Repeat with the first hand over and over. "Yoni" is the Sanskrit word for "vagina," and this move supposedly feels like he's entering a thousand different vaginas!

Again, these don't require an Olympic background in gymnastics to complete and are certainly an interesting twist on the same tired old handjob.

Don't feel as though you have to spend a lot of money to try something new. You may be a bit hesitant to drop a paycheck on a sex toy emporium, but you can definitely get kinky without having to spend a mint. For instance, common items around the house that can be used for a spanking scene involve spatulas, pans, spoons, or ping-pong paddles. You can try using a rolling pin to give massages. Heck, go into your laundry room while your dryer is set to tumble and take a tumble yourself on top of it!

Bring food into it! Food play is simple, sexy, and fun. Try covering your man in chocolate or whipped cream or pudding or anything you'd like to lick and then lick it off of him in lines. You can also feed chocolate-dipped fruit to each other. (The only thing to be careful of is sugary items around your vagina. If sugar gets into your vagina it becomes a prime breeding ground for yeast, which you definitely want to avoid.)

Try some light bondage. There are indeed people out there who are into their chains, but if those are just too intimidating for you, there are other, lighter ways to make it work. Consider using neckties or scarves to tie wrists or ankles together. If you're really nervous, you can just wrap them around your wrists and hold the ends of the ties in your hands. If you want to get into bondage a little more seriously but not spend a lot of money, consider investing in zip ties. They are virtually unbreakable and very inexpensive. (Just make sure to wrap a scarf or sock around body parts first so that the zip tie doesn't accidentally cut too much into the skin.)

Put on a show for your partner. Masturbating in front of your partner isn't just a way to turn him on, but it's also a great way to show him what you do when you're alone. After all, you definitely know what you like, right? Show your partner and you'll reap the benefits! It's also very educational for you as well to watch your man masturbate. And even if you've never thought of that being a sexy thing to watch, you may be surprised. You like to watch your man in pleasure when he's having sex with you, right? It's also fun to watch him in the throes of pleasure when he's going at it solo!

Consider toys. Again, they aren't necessary, but they *can* up your game to a whole other level. You don't need to go with giant rubber penises or massive vibrators, either. There are tons of much more discreet products to choose from if you're a bit hesitant. There is also a wide *array* of products for you to choose from, including things like Ben Wa balls or anal beads or cock rings. The options are literally endless so get on the internet and do some research. If you're not shy, you can go to your local sex shop and see what they have on display.

Share your fantasies with each other. As mentioned earlier in the book, if you feel hesitant to talk about your sexual fantasies with your partner, that's a bad sign. Additionally, just because you *talk* about your fantasies does not mean that you have to actually act them out. (And depending on the fantasy, fulfilling it may not be possible, anyway. Your man may have a thing for

20-armed tentacle monsters, but even if you were down with the same thing it would be rather hard to find a tentacle monster to play with.)

The simple act of sharing may turn you on and get you closer. Not to mention, simply talking about sex may be enough to make you hot.

Talk dirty to him. Most men love phone sex. Even if you're going to see each other later on tonight, there's no reason not to engage in a bit of afternoon delight with him on his lunch break. This will turn him on early in the day and keep you on his mind until he gets home at night. If you can't bring yourself to actually utter the words on the phone (or if you're in an area that is too public for dirty talk), send some sexy texts.

Consider sexy pictures. Many women aren't comfortable with sending nudes to their men, but men definitely love it when women do. So go find a room with favorable lighting and get your selfie on. Another great idea is to have your partner take pictures of you, or perhaps videotape having sex together. Men, in particular, are very visual creatures, so having lots of visual stimulation of you on hand is a sure way to get you into his mind.

Also considering asking *him* to send *you* some sexy pictures. This isn't as common, but most men are very happy to oblige!

Don't get scripted. Sex is wonderful when it's spontaneous! Make sure that you sometimes jump him when he gets out of the shower or right when he walks in the room. Many people get in the trap of scheduling their sex like it's an errand, rather than a true expression of love and affection. Keep your man guessing, and make it clear that you're open for unexpected advances on his part as well. This will keep your sex life fresh and exciting.

Consider investing in a book collection. Books like this can help you keep things exciting and give you ideas for when you get stuck in a rut. But don't feel as though you have to be consigned solely to advise books! Getting great sexual fantasy literature will give you great ideas as well.

Watch porn together. While many women don't exactly like visual pornography all that much, it's a rare man who does not. Even if you're not that into porn yourself, consider watching it with your man. He will likely find it an unbelievable turn on, and it may be a source of new ideas, just like your book collection is.

Don't get focused on the end goal. Even if you have the most amazing sex life in the world, both partners are not going to orgasm all the time. You may be under stress or your body just isn't feeling it that day for whatever reason. This can also happen with him - he's not a sex machine either. Don't be goal-oriented when it comes to sex; be experience-oriented. You can have an encounter where you, your man, or both you and your man do not orgasm and that doesn't make the sex bad.

Laugh. Sex is funny. You'll make funny noises and occasionally you'll be in the middle of a complicated move when he rolls over onto his car keys, gets poked in the ass, and loses his erection. It happens. Also, make sure to engage in playful acts that may not be directly sex-related. For instance, try buying body paint or playing strip Twister or something like that. This will keep your sex lives more fun, and create that environment of intimacy where both of you will be more inclined to trust and engage with the other.

Chapter 6 Communication Practices

The absolute greatest sex – by far – happens between two people who care about each other's pleasure equally and unselfishly.

If you want to have great sex, throw out your ego, throw out any self-absorption you have in your sex life, and throw out any sexual selfishness.

Communication must begin from a place of mutual caring for each other's pleasure and satisfaction, from a place of vulnerability, and most importantly, from a place of trust. Only from there can one's sex life reach astronomical heights.

Communication is harped on constantly in sex articles on the internet. But they rarely go farther than, "You should communicate with your partner about what you like and don't like, and be attentive to your partner's needs." While this is true, it goes much deeper than that.

Having sex is one of the most vulnerable acts you can do with another person. All of your insecurities, all of your anxieties, all of your stress about your performance, your body image, your past experiences – they can all converge in the bedroom.

When communicating with your partner, try your best to practice empathy. Try your best to put yourself in their shoes and see things from their perspective. And if they aren't doing this for you, let them know that you would like them to.

It's also important to set up boundaries in the bedroom, especially when you get deeper into sexual fantasies and the kinkier stuff. It takes a long time to build trust in one another, so that trust should be held sacred.

Here's a comment from a Redditor that applies to this topic:

"Trust in the bedroom builds up over time and can be taken away in a second. Define what trust means in and out of the bedroom."

And another Redditor talking about discussing sex with your partner:

"Also, I think that some people may experience awkwardness talking about sex. It's not always easy to discuss casually, we're so afraid of hurting people's feelings or feeling judged."

I think both of these comments hold true.

You may want to tell your partner that you don't like something they've been doing in bed for months, but you haven't had the heart to hurt their feelings. You have decided to keep it inside, but it's becoming a bigger and bigger issue for you. It's hard to bring these things up with someone you care about, and even more difficult to say it in a way that doesn't hurt their feelings.

You may also want to try something new, but this "something" has been deemed "weirder" by societal standards or is not as common, making you feel like you can't talk about it. But it has been eating away at your thoughts and your fantasies. You want to discuss trying it with your partner. You just don't know-how. You don't want them to judge you.

I have laid out exact scripts and worksheets you can use to work through this communication with your partner. I'm framing them in a letter format because going through dialogue wouldn't provide as good of an example.

You can use these as samples or follow them exactly. Either way, they should help ease the process. I have also included some helpful considerations to keep in mind when discussing these issues.

Script #1 – Discussing Something You Want to Try

There's something I've been meaning to talk to you about, but I've been holding off on it because it makes me feel a little uncomfortable. I'm more comfortable with you than I have been with anyone else, so I'm going to push through and say it anyway.

It's about something I've been wanting to try in the bedroom. It's not exactly something that our friends have done, and it makes me feel weird just thinking about it. But it has been eating away at my thoughts and I can't keep it in any longer. And most importantly, I want to try it with you, because I trust you so much and my feelings for you are so strong.

I want to try being handcuffed *(note: or whatever you want to try)*. I know you're not into being dominant, but I would love for you have total control over me in the bedroom, at least once, just to see how it is. If you do this for me, I would love to do something for you as well. It'll be like a trade!

Either way, if you are absolutely not comfortable with it, that is totally fine. I don't want you to feel pressured into it, and I wouldn't want to feel that way myself. But I do think it would be something fun to try. If we end up hating it, we can stop immediately. And if we end up loving it, awesome!

Let me know what you think.

Keep in mind-

- Your partner may be uncomfortable with what you want to try, so communicate that you understand this.
- Let them know this isn't something you want to do with just anyone, but that you want to share it with them and them alone (I get that this won't be totally true all the time, but it makes it more special).

- Try to see your request from your partner's perspective, and be empathetic to how they may feel about it.

- Don't pressure them. The more you pressure them, the easier it will be for them to deny your request and more conflict will arise. Give them a way out by saying if they're too uncomfortable, it's okay and it won't change the relationship.

- If your partner is making this type of request to you, imagine that you had a burning desire to try something. Step into your partner's shoes. Think about how you would want your partner to react. Then react accordingly.

Script #2 – Telling Your Partner That You Don't Like Something They Do in Bed

Our sex life is absolutely amazing. You're a freak in bed and you turn me on so much. I get horny just thinking about you as I go about my day.

I love everything you do in bed, especially when you pull my hips into you whenever we have sex *(or whatever you genuinely love about what they do)*. But there's just one thing that I know you like to do, and it's really hot, but it actually kind of hurts me *(or the reason why you don't like it)*.

I wish it didn't, but I can't control it. And I don't want you to feel bad thinking that it's your fault or anything. It's something neither of us can control.

When we're in that position where you're on top of me, and you roll your hips side to side, it feels really good for the most part, except it hurts my lower back quite a lot. I think it's from an old injury I got in high school, but it's pretty painful.

I don't mean to make you feel bad, because if it wasn't for my back, I would love it 100%. You look so hot when you're rolling your hips like that. But it hurts enough to where it totally distracts me from your sexiness.

I know I can't be a complete saint, so if there is anything I'm doing that you don't like, feel free to tell me. I'd rather both of us openly communicate like this and get these things out of the way, than stay silent doing things in the bedroom that actually hinder our sex life.

Keep in mind-

- Your partner may love doing the thing you don't like, and may think that you love it as well. If this is the case, some of their sexual ego and self-esteem may be tied to this act. So let them know the reason(s) why you don't like it, as gently as you can.

- Compliment them on the things you like first. Make them genuine comments. There's no use in communication if you are going to lie and fabricate things. Be honest, but be tactful in your honesty.

- Extend the lines of communication by being open to finding out something they don't like which you do in bed. This makes it more of an open forum, rather than one person being targeted.

Script #3 – Discussing a Fantasy You Have

This is something I have never shared with anyone. I only think about this when I am by myself, and I've kept it a secret for years.

But I want to share it with you because I trust you not to judge me, even if you don't want to try it.

I have this sexual fantasy. It feels weird for me to actually explain it out loud, so please, don't make fun of me. It's a fantasy where you knock on the front door and pretend like you're delivering a package *(insert whatever fantasy you have)*. We don't know each other, but when we see each other, we're immediately attracted to one another.

You say it's hot outside, so I invite you in for a drink. But next thing I know, you grab my face, pull it into yours, we start kissing, and eventually stumble into the bedroom and have sex.

I know it sounds a little funny, and it's not like I would want something like that to happen in real life. But I feel so comfortable with you, so pretending like we didn't know each other would be really hot for me.

How do you feel about it?

I also want you to feel comfortable telling me any fantasies you have that you would like to act out. We might as well get them all out in the open and see which ones we want to try. I think it could be really fun. What do you say?

Keep in mind-

- Fantasies can be uncomfortable to discuss, whether they are your own or your partner's. However, they are also completely natural. Pretty much everyone has them. So try to create an environment of understanding in which to let them out.
- Invite your partner to share their fantasies as well.

Script #4 – Talking About Your Insecurities and Anxieties

I wish this didn't bother me, but I can't help it. I feel really insecure about it and it makes me extremely anxious. It's got to do with something we do in the bedroom.

Up until now, I haven't said anything. I know I should have said something in the beginning, and that's my mistake, but I didn't want you to feel like I was taking something away from you. I also know that it's my insecurity and I have to deal with it myself, but it's gotten to a point where I can't do it anymore – at least not for a while until I work through it.

Using the dildo on you makes me very uncomfortable. It's bigger than me, and I'm scared you might like it more than me. I know this is crazy, because that thing is a piece of rubber. But I can't help it. Every time we use it, it makes me feel so uncomfortable.

I know that it's something you enjoy, and to think that a toy could replace me is nuts. But it's an insecurity I have been dealing with my whole life. I hope you can understand that.

I am totally open to other toys, so if there is something else you want to try in the meantime, I'm all ears. I just can't use that one anymore. I'll get through it eventually, but for now, it's causing me too much stress.

Thanks for being so understanding. If you have something you would like to talk about, I promise I won't judge you either and I'll do my best to help you through it.

Keep in mind-

- Insecurities run deep. They can cause people intense amounts of stress and anxiety, especially when it comes to sex.

- In the present, insecurities are largely uncontrollable. It takes time to work through these things. So if your partner suddenly brings up something they would like to stop doing in bed, don't take it personally. This may be something they have been dealing with for years, and it may have been hard to talk to you about it.

- Also, don't be afraid to express your insecurities. Often, one of the best ways to get through them is simply to let them out. Tell them to someone you trust and who cares about you. They may be able to provide a different perspective to help you out.

- Once again, maintain an open forum. When expressing an insecurity, your partner may be harboring their own. Give them an opportunity to express theirs as well so you can work through each other's together.

Establishing Boundaries

Knowing each other's boundaries is an essential part of communication. This is where you really get to know your partner's likes, dislikes, and subtle sexual tendencies. These play out in the bedroom constantly, so it's important that you're attentive to them.

I understand this is harder to do with casual relationships and one-night stands. Sometimes the nature of the relationship dictates that this stuff isn't communicated.

What you can do is a simplified version of what I'm about to show you. You would do everything verbally, and usually right after or right before having sex. Then, if you end up having sex again, you will understand much more about your partner's desires, your partner will understand much more about your own, and it will materialize itself into better sex.

I got this idea from a commenter on Reddit. The commenter noted that when she first got together with her partner of 10 years, she wrote out a list of things for them to discuss their sex life. Each item was rated on a scale of 1-10. Afterward, they could swap papers, compare answers, and have a much more open and structured discussion about their sex life.

They also came up with a sexual bucket list, which can give partners goals to strive for and make trying new things more fun. I think both of these ideas are brilliant.

Using these two ideas, you can gain a number of things:

- Knowledge of what your partner likes and dislikes.
- What boundaries you should stick to.
- A platform for open communication.

- Goals to work towards together.
- A way to communicate without actually having to say anything, which can make it easier to get started.

I've come up with two sample lists, one including topics for discussion where you would provide a rating for each, and another with possible goals for a sexual bucket list.

I suggest using these as a guide, creating your own, and trying them out. You never know how much it could deepen your connection and improve your communication skills.

Topics for discussion (the first four came from the Redditor)-

1. What level of trust do you have for your partner in the bedroom?
2. How kinky are you?
3. How kinky do you think your partner is?
4. How kinky are you willing to go for your partner?

5. How comfortable are you talking openly about sex?

6. How much do you enjoy giving oral sex?

7. How much do you enjoy receiving oral sex?

8. How much foreplay do you like, 1 being "not very much" and 10 being "a lot"?

9. How willing are you to try anal sex?

10. How willing are you to try having sex in public?

11. How willing are you to try experimenting with sex toys?

12. How comfortable do you feel with being vocal in the bedroom?

13. How comfortable do you feel being constrained by your partner?

14. How comfortable do you feel being blindfolded?

15. How comfortable do you feel watching porn with your partner?

16. How comfortable are you discussing sexual fantasies?

17. How comfortable are you acting out sexual fantasies?

18. How much do you enjoy being more dominant?

19. How much do you enjoy being more submissive?

20. How much do you struggle with sexual anxiety and insecurity?

When you print it out, write a number from 1 to 10 next to each question. Each partner should fill out their own answer sheet.

Afterward, switch papers and read over your partner's answers. Then discuss each answer. Along the way, you will figure out where your partner's boundaries lie and where to go from there.

Example Sexual Bucket List-

- Have sex on the beach
- Perform oral sex while driving
- Have sex in the backseat of a car
- Have sex on the kitchen floor

- Use a toy on each other at the same time
- Take a trip to the sex shop together
- Watch porn together
- Play a sexual card game
- Have sex four times in one day (or as many as you desire)
- Have sex in the shower
- Perform/receive oral sex in the shower
- Have sex with the curtains open
- Have sex while watching a movie
- Read an erotic book together
- Try constraining each other
- Fulfill one fantasy of each partner
- Research tantric sex together
- Try five new positions every month
- Have anal sex
- Surprise one another with a sexual gift
- Add multitasking into the bedroom
- Have a threesome

- Try switching dominant and submissive roles
- Have sex in every room of the house
- Have sex every day for a month straight
- Have morning sex every day before work for a month straight
- Have sex while cooking dinner
- Have sex while eating dinner
- Make a porno together

Each partner would create their own, switch with their partner, then collaborate with each other on what they want to pursue.

Applying the Communication Principles

The biggest part of communication is practicing empathy. You have to try your best to see where your partner is coming from, and they should do the same for you.

The next big thing is being open and honest with your partner. It's okay if you feel uncomfortable. These things are inherently uncomfortable, **but that's why it is so important to talk about them.**

Bottling up these thoughts and feelings doesn't do you any good.

Expressing them does you a world of good and will bring you and your partner closer together. You may also experience some of the craziest sex of your life. And all you had to do was tell your partner you wanted to try something new.

Communicate with empathy, communicate honestly and openly, establish boundaries, and write out your desires.

Ba da bing, ba da boom. Great sex awaits.

Chapter 7 Forgetting About Past Ghosts

We all sometimes think about the past for different reasons; it is completely normal to think about it, and sometimes, it is even inevitable. However, there is a point where we need to stop thinking about it so much or avoid doing it all together. That is when it keeps bringing us bad memories that are preventing us from enjoying our present and preventing us from moving on.

When positive things come to our mind, thinking about past experiences doesn't bring any negative effects; but when these thoughts tend to come with any signs of sadness, anger or distress, it might be better to leave them buried in time. It is important to remember that the unpleasant experiences we had are now behind us and even if they hurt at the time, we cannot let them hurt us forever. The truth is that bad things happen to everyone. Some of these things are worse than others, and some are harder to forget; but it is important to move on without letting those experiences drag us down. If we constantly let our memories haunt us, then we are the ones sabotaging ourselves. There is no doubt that sometimes our past can affect our present and our future, and that is why we need to cut those chains, and you are the only one that can do that. Nobody else but ourselves can control our minds and thoughts so slowly, but surely we need to train ourselves to block those things that come with repercussions.

There are many things from the past that can affect us. These are the most common ones: past experiences, past comments, or people. All of these things have the potential to affect us significantly and in some cases, it is hard to just let these things go. Sometimes it is difficult, and you might think it is impossible to let whatever that is affecting you go, but we need to do it, sometimes all together or sometimes step by step. And the first step is to understand how much your life can improve if you don't focus on these pasts ghosts. If we let these things bother us constantly, they can affect our self-esteem, the ability to trust, our relationships with others, our plans, and many other things. You might not think it is that important or that deep, but whatever that is negative can affect you somehow. So you need to find a way to move away from that in order to have good relationships with others and with yourself.

We are going to be focusing on the times that past ghosts affect our emotional, physical and sexual life. If your relationship is being affected by something from the past, there are two possibilities. (A) What is affecting you is related to an experience you went through while in the relationship. Something that your significant other did or said that ended up hurting you and caused issues in the relationship. (B) Something that happened in the past that is not related to your partner but still manages to affect your relationship. Whether your case is A or B, you need to know that you are not the only person that has ever been affected by any of these; luckily, it is never too late to try to move forward.

Being affected by something that happened during our marriage

Marriages are complex; they are full of ups and downs. Therefore, there is going to be more than one occasion that has certain experiences that hurt to remember. We need to consider something, however. If you are still with someone, it is because you decided to be with them regardless of anything else that might have happened between the two of you. If you decided to forgive your spouse because of something they said/did, then you need to try to get over that dark experience. Basically, you need to forgive and forget. It is not enough with you doing the first one, you need to try and do the two of them. We understand that forgetting something, especially something painful is not that simple, and the truth is we might not be able to forget about it completely because it might still run through our head from time to time. However, we need to stop giving it importance. Don't spend any time thinking about it. Any time that this bad memory pops up, you need to eradicate it, and think about something good instead. Even if it's still in your mind, try not to speak about it. Constantly bringing up the past can be equally damaging to a relationship. When you are trying to construct something positive, you don't need a constant reminder of the negative things. This is bad for both parties; the other person will constantly feel accused and they will eventually feel like every attempt is in vain, and that no matter how hard they try to amend things, they will always be attacked because of the past. Also, the person who is bringing it up will never be able to get healed and will start exhibiting toxic behaviors in the relationship, even though in their head, they think they are the victims. Whether what happened between you and your partner was something big or small, pointing fingers forever, especially after coming to an agreement to try to fix things, is very unhealthy. If the actions that hurt you are small issues, then think that it is not worth to bring your relationship down for something that is meaningless. If your relationship was affected by something more serious, the fact that both of you decided to overcome it and keep trying, speaks a lot. If you didn't let adversity break you down, do not let past memories do so.

Being affected by something that happened outside or before our marriage

It is common to be haunted by painful memories that happened before/outside our marriage, or things that don't have anything to do with your spouse, but still somehow affect our relationship. Things that cause us great pain, no matter how deep into the past they are, can still manage to affect different aspects of our lives; but we need to let those things go for our own good and for the good of people around us. We deserve to be happy and not let anybody or anything that is no longer relevant still take a toll on our well-being. If you keep bringing these things up and bringing insecurities into your life, this is going to affect your relationship with others as well, including your relationship with your spouse. You can count on your spouse to help you, and that is absolutely fine. Be honest with your spouse. Let them know about those things that affect you, and ask them to help you leave those issues behind. Couples are there to support each other, and facing things together is the best way to overcome problems. What is not okay, however, is to blame our spouse for things they are not guilty of. As an example, let's say that in the past you were with a partner that was unfaithful to you and now you think that your current partner will also be unfaithful even if they have done nothing to make you believe this. You can't just assume that everybody's the same. Just because someone said or did something, doesn't mean someone else is going to do it as well. You cannot put everybody into the same category. Your spouse is not guilty or responsible for the things that you might have experienced in the past, so why hold grudges against them? Past events sometimes bring insecurities, and it is understandable; but attacking people because of your insecurities is not alright. Do not forget that sometimes, instead of judging others, we need to judge ourselves. We have all the right to be happy, so don't be the one who is actually getting on the way.

The ways those past ghosts can affect your relationship

- You hold anger towards your significant other for something that happened between the two of you in the past.

- You cannot stop thinking about the negative experiences from the past.

- Bad thoughts related to past experiences are preventing you from expressing yourself the way you would like to sexually/romantically.

- You feel that you cannot forgive your significant other for something they did/said.

- You can't trust people, including your significant other, for something someone else did/said.

- You constantly victimize yourself.

- You are stuck to the past.

- You don't believe people can change.

If you identify yourself with one of the problems mentioned above, then it's most than likely that your relationship is currently being affected by past grudges. We have previously spoken about the reasons why you might be feeling this way, and the importance of not letting things get in the way, as well as how to stop them from doing so. However, we understand that sometimes, things are not that easy to see; but even if you only suspect that your relationship is being affected, it is good to put the things you learned into practice. You don't have to wait until things aggravate more. In fact, the sooner you tackle a problem, the better.

The moment something gets in the way of you being able to enjoy your emotional, physical, and sex life with plenitude, it is the moment you need to consider this as a problem. It is not fair for us or for our spouse to prevent ourselves from living the kind of relationship we would like to have, just because we cannot move on.

Having a relationship is easy, but in order to have a healthy and strong relationship, the people involved have to work hard and be able to enjoy every aspect of the relationship.

The ghost of previous relationships and experiences

We all have a past and it is completely normal to have had a romantic and a sexual life before being with the person you're currently with. We can't deny what had happened, but that does not mean we have to constantly bring it up. Many relationships suffer from a very unpleasant problem of having to constantly hear about exes, deal with them or even worse, being compared to them.

It is not okay to compare people; it is disrespectful and it can cause harm, although some people don't seem to understand that. They think that doing so is completely innocent, but the truth is that even if your partner doesn't say anything to you, having to hear explicit details about your romantic or sexual life with someone else is never easy and it can be very off-putting. Even if your partner is a laid-back type of person who is not jealous and whom you feel that you can talk to about anything, they still have feelings. You need to think before you speak. How would you feel if the situation was the other way around? At the end of the day, we can't read minds, and if you are constantly speaking about a person you were with before, that might set off some red alerts in your partner and bring some insecurities since they might feel you still think too much about somebody else, or still focusing on the past.

There are two scenarios when it comes to exes, you might still talk to them or you might not. If your ex is no longer part of your life, then let it go. Focus on the new chapter of your life, and focus on the special person that is now with you. On the other hand, if your ex is still part of your life, for whatever reason, maybe for personal choice or because of an obligation, then you need to draw a line. Your ex is not the person you are with; they are not your partner anymore. They are not the main priority in your life and you don't have to base your life decisions around them or let them interfere with your personal life. Even if your ex is a good friend of yours and someone you care for, they sometimes can overstep, so for the good of your new relationship, you must not let your ex interfere even if you think they are doing it in a good way. You and only you have got to decide what to do with your life, and letting exes get in the way might potentially damage your relationship. You are not obligated to cut contact with your previous partners. However, you must understand that the treatment between an ex and your spouse can't be the same. You must be patient and considerate with your significant other and understand why they might feel uncomfortable about your ex.

As we previously mentioned, sometimes people tend to compare their spouses with an ex or a previous partner and this can be very distasteful. We would recommend that you refrain from comparing, especially, if the comparison has to do with anything physical or sexual. Some people might think it is okay to compare especially if what they have to say favors their spouse; however, your point might come across better if you don't bring other people to the equation. There are other better ways to compliment someone. Try to do it in a way that will make your partner feel like they're the only person that you think about in that manner. Also, do not expect your partner to act the same way or do the same things that any of your previous romantic/sexual partners did. They are their own person and should not be held to previous expectations.

Be careful with expectations

Sometimes people have an idea of what being in a relationship is supposed to be like or how sex is supposed to be. Often, this idea is based on past experiences; things we have heard from others and even certain things such as the sexual content made available through the media. However, every relationship is different, and every person has their own interests and way of doing things. Your marriage is a unique experience in all of its branches and that includes sexual matters. Not everything that you hear from others would necessarily apply to you; have it in mind that if you hear it from someone else, that is from their own perspective and their criteria, which might be totally different from yours. Also, not everything you see from certain sexual content is realistic or accurate. So enjoy what you have, and if your sex life needs improvements, do it based on the needs and desires of the two of you. Have it in mind that the sexual content you see has a purpose, which is the purpose of entertaining. The people you see through that screen are after all doing a job; they have something to sell. They are not going to show you the not so glamorous parts of sex. Sexual content often does not equal what it is like to have sex in real life. If you are not comparing yourself to the people you see performing these acts, why comparing or expecting your partner to be like that, or to do what they do? Whether you watch this kind of content or not is completely up to you; many people do, some others don't. Nevertheless, if you are a viewer, it is okay to inspire yourself from certain things, but do not expect your sexual act to be exactly as you see it in a movie. Don't forget what reality is like. It is actually more common than it seems to hear people saying that addiction to sexual content has taken a toll, not only on their sex lives, but on their general well-being. Do not let other things interfere with your getting pleasure through actual contact, and between you and your loved ones.

The moment you make the relationship all about the two of you only, the moment that relationship will start blossoming.

Chapter 8 Loving Words Heal Relationships

The most dominant two phrases that heal a harmed relationship are additionally the two phrases that are hardest to state... "I'm Sorry" and "I was wrong"...This is basic in healing relationships for couples.

The motivation behind why these phrases are hardest to state is because we would prefer not to admit that we have caused whatever broke or harmed a relationship. More often than not, we say that it was the other person's deficiency. Also, we hang tight for that person to be the first to apologize. In any case, the apology never comes because the other person is likewise hanging tight for it.

What's more, we realize that relationships inside the family and outside of it sometimes end in light of the absence of this apology. We know many separations happen just because either never made a move to apologize.

For what reason is it so difficult to admit that we weren't right and to apologize? It is straightforward... that is human instinct, a shortcoming which puts us over the others. What we need is to defeat this commitment to self. This requires personal development, compassion, and thinking about the other. What's more, a necessary apology will reestablish that broken relationship.

It doesn't make a difference who fouled up when a relationship is broken. Significantly, we venture out. Remember that the other person feels a similar way. We should state something that can prompt healing, for example, "I'm sorry that we are having this issue. Would we be able to discuss making things right once more?"

Making a stride like this quite often prompts healing a broken relationship. Furthermore, more often than not, the conversation results in the two gatherings saying 'sorry,' and this typically leads in a more grounded relationship.

Any healing in a relationship for couples requires some forgiveness. This should originate from the heart before it is said in words.

One must be cautious about is that as it may, in communicating forgiveness. To state "I forgive you" amidst a battle may be misjudged as "You weren't right," and would compound the situation. We should say "I forgive you" just when the other person requests forgiveness. At that point, these become the ideal words. Mercy can heal the relationship as well as the bodies and the brains of the two persons.

Keep in mind, in healing relationships for couples, we as of now have the words. We need to state them.

Have an incredible relationship by utilizing words that heal

FALLING IN LOVE - THROUGH YOUR OWN LOVE WORDS

Regardless of whether you have begun to look all starry eyed at years prior, or hoping to become hopelessly enamored now, I can share with you some extremely sentimental approaches to share your emotions. Purchasing a love card, or a romantic ballad is excellent, in any case, words mean more when you get them directly from your own heart. You need to realize how to state what you might want to express. From that point forward, applying some inventiveness will make you incline that your beginning to look all starry eyed at just because.

- Address it with the right "pet name."
- Use detail, and don't be hesitant to get "mushy."
- Express yourself enthusiastically with love quotes
- Be inventive and unique include something new.

When writing to the love of your life, it is great to start it off with a pet name. Perhaps you have something that nobody else hears? This would be the ideal time to use it. This love letter will be among you and the one you love, so make it individual. A few people like to use (infant, sweetie, hun, and so on). I state if you have something nobody thinks about because it might be excessively humiliating this is the time to use it.

When writing a sentimental love letter, it is tied in with being mushy. Express yourself now with all the soft stuff that you typically don't state. Try not to keep down, after this is the thing that a love letter is about. Get energetic with your words, and let that individual recognize what your heart feels for them.

Presently, someplace in the middle of the letter, use their real name. You would prefer not to overdo it by a considerable amount of pet names, yet one to start, and real name in the middle ought to be great. Make sure to use love quotes all through this gem. Genuine romance does not come around over and over again. You need to make sure you treat it well and care for it while you have it. You're telling them you love them, with imaginative detail.

Include something new. Something you have not raised in quite a while, or at no other time. Demonstrate to them that something new emerges to you. State what your heart needed to shout, the day you realized you were in love. Connections can be precarious, yet if you enable yourself to recollect how much you are in love, you will do fine.

How to Express Love Words

Communicating with a person that you genuinely like them calls for the use of love words. Love is the single component that makes a society what it is. Without love, there is no life, and this is the motivation behind why words of love are significant. There are numerous things that best display love words, and when the name is referenced, many recognize what it implies. People use multiple ways and incorporate the words and, they can do it orally, or they can write it down. The vast majority when they were growing up, they used to write love letters to one another. Today, people keep on composing love letters. This is an instrument used to display love words. It is a rare occurrence natural to impart these words, and it calls for certified fondness. There is something men do that best express the words. Initially, understand that words are simply words if there is no activity to coordinate. This is likely the best thing about love. Love is best shown in any case when words are included. It affirms what there as of now is.

In this manner, if you wish to use the words, it is vital that you reexamine yourself and see if you love the person. Sentimental love between a man and a lady is the thing that I have portrayed above and a portion of the words that you will discover incorporate the accompanying. Dear sweetheart, nectar, my love, my dearest, and the list goes on. Love is dynamic, and people are inventive. New ages keep on concocting love words like baby, boo, and numerous others. When it comes to utilizing these words, it is vital that you ensure that the person you are communicating to gets it. When there is viable correspondence, you can likewise anticipate just useful things in your relationship. There are such vast numbers of love words that you can use and different societies, and even religions may decide the words. Different dialects will have their one of a kind arrangement of words. While you wish to express your love to somebody, it doesn't need to be sexual love. You can have respect for your children, guardians, sisters, etc. It is additionally extremely vital to express appreciation to such people, and many do it consistently.

Coming up are next to a portion of the words that people use to demonstrate their children love pumpkin, bear, love bear, daylight, baby, and the list goes on. You can think of your one of a kind words which can be a nickname at the same time, is equipped with love. It is important to be active in showing love to other people. In society, some people frequently feel dismissed. Such people might not have dear companions or family. Life is desolate when you have nobody to impart to and you ought to endeavor to make love any place and whenever conceivable. If you're the sort of person who isn't active in showing love, begin doing as such, and you don't need to write a love letter. It is the thing that you state and how you state it. Love can include numerous viewpoints and figure out how to radiate through your cooperative attitude.

Using Words of Love to Inspire the Relationship - 3 Tips for Men to Learn

Cherishing Love Inspires the Heart to Create Words that Gives Love its Life.

Relationships are a back and forth movement on the life of all of us as we clear our path through the riddles of life and of love. To live in the steady "fight," as some are inclined to call it, is to live in the bogus acknowledgment that in one way or another there are always victors and failures as we cross the minefield of love.

I come at it from an altogether different point of view as I take a gander at the words, we as a whole appear to use to get us to where we even have a relationship. Men, generally, need such a considerable amount of assistance in this field and typically wallow because of poor role models, societal impacts, peer pressure and only by and large sluggishness in needing to be something more with their words to their partner.

There is always a way out, yet numerous men neglect to search for the way in any case when it comes to talking love to their partner.

So, what are a few ways to make words mean things again with your partner? A couple of tips can always prove to be useful, right men?

Tip 1: Women need to hear your heart. Most likely one of the hardest things for men to do as a result of the reality they were never educated how to do as such. Begin little here, folks — an all-around set note left before work can be an incredible begin. The significant thing to do here is to claim your powerlessness to share your heart NOW yet disclose to her that you are learning.

Tip 2: Not each cherishing word should lead to sex! What a stun man. Because you state something decent doesn't imply that the spoken words are S-E-X! Get over yourself. In some cases, the most sentimental things we do will never lead to sex, nor should they.

Tip 3: Love to love. Reevaluate your relationship as a way to love simply cherishing your partner. If you center around the quintessence of your identity as a team, the relationship will rule your faculties.

Keep in mind, men. You are more than what you at any point, though you were with your words. Presently, live that way.

At last, Love is All There is So Let Your Words be Your Beginning.

Chapter 9 What Women Want; What Men Want

Since men and women are wired differently, how they approach sex also differs. There are a number of things that both of them want, but they may not explicitly express the desire for such things, for one reason or the other. Partners should always remember to communicate and to always think of their partners' feelings.

Things Women Want:

- **Threesomes**

One of the surprising things that women want is threesomes. Usually, it is men who are supposed to be keen on having a threesome. However, many women have been known to have had fantasies about having a threesome with another female.

It is important to point out that even though some people may have such fantasies, not every one of them would find the fantasies as pleasurable if the couple decided to play out some of these fantasies out in real life.

Couples should also note that threesomes may complicate the relationship. They can lead to feelings of jealousy and insecurity from either of them. It is advisable to seek someone who is not close to any of you if you choose to walk down that path.

- **Role-Playing**

Women crave adventure, especially where romance and sex are concerned. Women are therefore more imaginative. Roleplay is one of the ways couples can spice up their sex lives, by using their imagination to maximize the sexual experience between them.

Role play is one of the best ways to break a sex life that has become routine. It adds a fresh approach to sex and creates a sense of excitement that both couples have not felt for some time.

You can add costumes to make the roles more authentic. Some women may want to be dominated, while others want to experience the feeling of being in control. However, if you chose to do it, both parties must always feel comfortable with the roles they play, otherwise it will not work.

- **Sex Toys**

Couples are encouraged to use sex toys, particularly when the woman cannot get orgasms when she is with her partner. There are sex toys that are specifically designed for couples.

- **Rough sex**

Some studies have shown that 57% of women love it a little bit rough in the bedroom. Most women who would love rough sex, like to play a submissive role. The intensity of it may vary, depending on the woman.

Some women like a little bit of roughness like grabbing her from the waist pulling her tightly towards you. Others may want an even more intense experience that may qualify as S&M. it is therefore advisable that couples talk about what makes either of them uncomfortable, before trying out new things in the bedroom.

Some commentators and writers have pointed out that some women may be reluctant to rough sex, because it may contradict feminism and women empowerment. Despite the fact that they fantasize about it, they feel it may undermine their position as an equal in a relationship.

However, nothing can be further from the truth. Rough sex, in this case, is more like role-playing. Taking a submissive position in the bedroom should not mean that you are less than your partner. In any case, many powerful men have for centuries sought out dominatrix in brothels, in order to gain pleasure from this submissive position they assume.

What Men Want:

There are a few things men fantasies about. As stated earlier, they are often simple and direct. Despite the fact that these things seem simple and physical, they can go a long way in helping you get to new levels of excitement.

- **Initiate Sex**

Men find it very flattering when a woman initiates sex. It is generally expected that men would initiate sex. For that reason, many men secretly wish their wives would initiate sex. It excites men on several levels. One is compliments and reassures him that he is wanted and it makes him feel attractive.

It is surprising and exciting when the woman suddenly initiates sex. It does not have to be complicated. Simply making a move and expressing your desire either verbally or physically will be appreciated by most guys.

- **Try New Positions**

Just like initiating sex, it can be a real turn-on for him when she initiates new things in the bedroom. Some women have reservations about making this kind of move. They feel he may take it like she is cheating or that she is saying that he is not good enough in bed.

However, most mature men appreciate when the woman takes the initiative. Many men out there also find it somewhat flattering that she is keen on trying new positions with him in the bedroom.

- **Watching Her**

Men respond much more to visual stimuli than women do. Men are easily aroused by a woman dancing provocatively in front of him. She may also choose to touch herself in front of him, especially if this is something that also turns her on.

- **Compliments**

Men have an ego and this is also true when it comes to sex. Giving him compliments that say something about his skills is not only beneficial to him, but it can be helpful to the woman as well. There are many other things you can compliment him on, including his fit body, charm, or masculinity.

Chapter 10 Tips to Have More Intimacy in Every Situation

There are many ways to spice up your sex life, and as you learned there is a lot beyond the bedroom that can be done to enhance it as well. This chapter will explore some ideas of what you can do to make your sex life even better outside of the bedroom.

Do Fun Things Together

Doing fun things together allows you to increase your dopamine levels together as well. When you have fun together, it increases your closeness with one another and can enhance the joy you experience with each other. It adds a unique sense of intimacy to your relationship that cannot be added by sexual experiences.

Ideally, you want to have fun together in a way that gets your blood pumping and your adrenaline rushing. Going to an amusement park, ice skating, visiting an upbeat concert, or otherwise doing something fun and exciting can increase the happiness of your experience with one another.

Having fun this way can add energy to your relationship that will carry into the bedroom and make sex even more enjoyable.

Kiss More Often

Many couples, especially those who have been together a while tend to kiss less often. Kissing is a highly romantic and passionate act and should be done regularly. Think about it, at the beginning of the relationship you likely kissed your partner a lot more frequently than you do now that you are more comfortable together. You want to start doing it more often.

When you are kissing more regularly, don't just increase the volume but also increase the passion in each kiss. There is no need to peck and go. Give the kiss a few moments and truly experience your partner with each kiss. You can include your hands and body as well, or even kiss in other intimate areas such as on the cheek, forehead or hand.

Recall What It Was Like to Meet

When you first met you likely spent a lot more time getting to know one another and a lot less time watching TV or doing other things to pass the time. You can spend some time asking each other questions about life, or even just reminisce on the days when you met each other. Getting to know each other all over again is a great way to rekindle the flame in a relationship.

The reality is that we don't all stay the same in life. Throughout your relationship, you and your partner will change several times over. Their preferences for certain things may change, and these are all great things to learn about each other all over again as you rekindle your love by communicating and asking questions.

Describe Your Sexual Fantasies

Many times, sex is just about the act and couples don't really speak a lot about sex outside of the bedroom. A great way to spark up a flame and add passion to your sex life is to talk about each other's fantasies and interests. This gives you an opportunity to get to know each other's sexual preferences more intimately which means that you can gain maximum enjoyment out of sex. It allows you to have a better idea of what your partner likes and what they don't like, and how you can make sexual experiences more enjoyable for them.

Keep the Mystery Alive

In relationships, it can be easy to get to know each other so intimately that there appears to be no mystery left in the relationship anymore. This can be counterproductive to the process of bringing romance back into your relationship. A lot of romance builds around mystery and the desire to know each other more intimately than you presently do. There are many ways that you can add mystery back into your relationship, even if you already know almost everything about each other. Using sentences that add mystery, clothes that spark intrigue and even simple texts that make the other partner wonder what you have planned for the evening can help add mystery back into the relationship.

When the mystery is present, the other person wonders about you. They start thinking about you and may even become obsessed with wanting to know what you have planned because they are curious. Curiosity is the key to creating mystery and getting your partner wondering about you and what you have to offer them that is unique from before.

Express Gratitude

A great way to help your partner feel cared for and show them how much they mean to you is to express your gratitude. Expressing gratitude takes very little time but can have a significant impact on the quality of your relationship. When people feel cared for and loved, they want to show more care and love to the one they feel for as well. This can increase the quality of your relationship, making you both feel more appreciated.

In relationships, the little things often get overlooked. People forget that the little things count and so they don't take the time to show appreciation and gratitude for them genuinely. Something as simple as "I really appreciate that you always support me in my decisions" or "I really appreciate that you make me breakfast each morning" can go a long way. Even though repeat activities can lead to things being expected, it is always good to show that you don't necessarily expect things to be done for you or in a certain way. Always show that you care about what your partner does in life and for you, as this will increase the quality of your time together and make you both feel more loved overall. When you feel more loved, the sparks will naturally fly in your relationship.

Don't Hold Grudges

Holding grudges can destroy relationships really quickly. When people hold grudges, they fail to let go of things that are no longer relevant, and it can lead to destruction in the relationship. You may feel that if you let go, it shows your partner that their mistake was acceptable, and for you, it may seem like you are allowing them to do it again. In reality, when you let it go, you are giving them permission to be human and make mistakes. It allows them the opportunity to see what they've done and make a change, knowing that you will appreciate the change wholeheartedly. It never pays to hold a grudge in your relationship.

Care About Self Care

How you care about yourself and how your partner cares about themselves is important when it comes to having a healthy relationship. A healthy relationship almost always leads to a healthy sex life, since your sex life is so closely linked to the health of your relationship. It is important that you both emphasize self-care and take the time to truly nurture your own needs before nurturing your partner's. Yes, before. You cannot pour out of an empty cup, and keeping your cup empty is not a favor to your partner. Instead, it is a drawback that will lead to your relationship falling apart.

Taking care of your own self can come in many ways. You should look towards developing a healthy relationship with yourself if you want to really get serious about self-care. Take yourself on dates, have alone time, and get to know yourself more. The added benefit of getting to know yourself more is that you learn things about yourself that you may not have known before. You can share these things with your spouse, thus expanding your realm of conversation topics and letting you continue to get to know each other, even long after the relationship has worn out its honeymoon phase.

There are many ways that you can spark romance back into your relationship outside of the bedroom. By having these types of activities present in your day-to-day life, you increase the amount of romance and intimacy that lies between you and your partner and it causes you both to become more eager about your sex life. A relationship that is rich outside of the bedroom is one that will be exciting inside of the bedroom.

When you are looking to cause sparks outside of the bedroom, you want to take your time and really get to know one another. Forget everything you've learned up until now and take the time to learn again. In many cases what you know now can be relevant but may no longer be the whole truth. People regularly change, and this can lead to there being a disconnection between what you are thinking and what your partner is wanting. By communicating, you can alleviate this disconnection and create a renewed sense of appreciation and romance between yourself and your partner.

Overall, the best thing you can do for your sex life is to nurture all areas of your relationship. The more successful your relationship is elsewhere, the more exciting your sex life will be. It creates a sense of deep knowing and trust that cannot be faked between two people. When this trust and love is present, the sex you experience will be unlike anything you have ever had before. Even relationships that have been alive for a long time can benefit from this type of rekindling.

Chapter 11 Restoring Intimacy in Your Marriage

No marriage is complete without intimacy. Intimacy is what brings spark and fire to a marriage. Intimacy leads to romance and romance is what entangles you two, turning two souls into one. Yes, this unification of your souls and bodies is what this next step is about and exactly what has been missing out in your dull marital life for a very long time. When you don't spend time together, the intimacy greatly reduces and without intimacy in a marriage, it is really hard to have a successful marriage. Therefore, to make your married life happy again, you need to bring back the 'intimacy' element in it. Here's how you can do that.

Focus on Your Appearance

To be intimate with your spouse, you need to entice them and for that, you need to look good. How long has it been since you focused on yourself? Take a good look at yourself in the mirror and you'll find out why your better half isn't attracted to you anymore. Yes, being into looks is something shallow, but good looks are what attract people. You become attracted to good-looking people and the same goes for your spouse too. So, if you want to seduce them, you need to dress up nicely, work on your hair and face and look your best.

Additionally, start exercising to shed off the few extra pounds you have gained. Most women don't want a pot-bellied man and most men would not want a woman with love handles. Furthermore, most people who are overweight have a low self-esteem and if you don't feel good about yourself, then you are unlikely to enjoy intimacy. Once you start making an effort towards looking better, your spouse will notice this and this is likely to re-ignite that spark and remind your spouse of the person they fell in love with.

Make a Happy Ritual

Experts say that most couples become so lost in their professional lives that they fail to make time for one another. They come home exhausted from work, rest a little, play with kids probably, eat something and go to bed to prepare themselves for another hectic day at work. This pretty much sums up their routine lives and when they eventually have time on the weekend, they just want to catch up on some more sleep. When they have no time for one another, the closeness between them slips away. However, in order to restore your marriage and bring back intimacy, it is critical to make time for one another and develop a happy ritual just for the two of you. A happy ritual refers to a ritual you and your spouse practice with each other at least once a day, so that you can find some time even if it is just for a few minutes to spend with your loved one.

For instance, a psychology teacher who experienced the same problem with his wife once created a happy ritual with his wife wherein the two danced on seeing one another. This gesture expressed their happiness on seeing one another and also helped them get a break from their monotonous routine. You could do something like this too or come up with a creative happy ritual wherein you both show your contentment for each other. You could sing songs to each other, or give each other big smiles, or say something beautiful to one another whenever you see each other after a long day at work.

Send Sexy Messages/Emails

You may have been together for quite some time; hence, you don't think that there is a need to send sex messages. However, this is where you are wrong. Do you remember when you first started dating? You would probably send sexy and interesting messages that you both looked forward to and you would not wait to see each other again and probably act out those fantasies. If you want to bring that spark back into your marriage then you had better consider sexting. Sexting is fun, thrilling, and exciting and by the time you see each other in the evening you are all excited and you know what happens from there. I know it can be hard but just start slowly and build up to sexting and you will be amazed at what it can do for your marriage.

Physical Contact

Expert psychologists say that a touch by someone you love can rekindle a spark inside you, which is why they advise their clients coming in for marriage counseling to touch each other often throughout the day, so their bodies become familiar with each other once again and they become tempted to explore each other further once more. Touching the arm, a light rub on the neck, or a pat on the legs are playful touches that can help you and your spouse bring back intimacy into your relationship. Make sure to do it more often, so your spouse knows you want them to come closer to you. Soon, they will start becoming playful with you as well.

Go on Dates

There was some time in your life when you and your spouse used to go on dates frequently. However, things aren't the same as before, but they can be. By simply doing what you guys did before, you can save your marriage. Make each other feel special by going on dates frequently. Surprise them with a candlelit dinner and then a serene walk by the beach. Treat them to a romantic picnic on the weekend or take them to a local but good bed and breakfast for a romantic day out. Make sure to keep everything romantic and smooth on your date and try not to bring up an upsetting topic or talk about kids, work and other responsibilities. Just be in the moment and enjoy each other's company and you will be amazed at what this can do for you.

Don't Set Limits

Once things start improving between the two of you after practicing the tips outlined in this book, you need to take care of one thing. Never set limits on what time and how many times you guys should spend time together and have sex. Be intimate and do whatever you feel whenever you feel like. Never stop your spouse from coming close to you because it's daytime or because you just did it. Just enjoy each other's company and closeness and celebrate the love you have because setting limits takes away freedom from you and this makes your life monotonous and exhausting.

Also, plan something special for your date nights. You could decorate the room with candles, or put on some romantic music to set up the mood and make your spouse drawn towards you.

Lots of interesting tips, right? Now, it is your job to implement them, so things become smooth and amazing for you and your better half once more.

Chapter 12 Tantric Sex For Marriage

When you begin to follow the path of tantric sex, you begin to find a change in yourself. You find yourself changing how you view yourself and how you view the world. You find yourself looking at relationships that will last a lifetime. Through your journey, you will learn that every man and woman has a certain level of divinity in them. You will start to view sex as a sacred act instead of just a physical act. You will also learn to love deeper and find that you are soaring to different levels of bliss.

You will only have a successful journey when you relieve yourself from any preconceived notions. You should not think of what you need to do and what your lover must do to please you. When you read this chapter, you will be able to identify new ideas about yourself and also embrace new ideas about yourself. You will also learn how to have great sex!

You will learn the basic concepts of tantric sex and identify new exciting ways to life and love. This chapter will be worth it!

The Yin and the Yang: Which is male and which is female?

You must be familiar with the stereotypes that men are from Mars and women are from Venus. This implies that men are assertive and extremely powerful while women are soft and fragile who are only fit for nurturing. There are other stereotypes that men do not show any feelings whatsoever, while women have a plethora of emotion that is ready to unleash itself in a second. It has also been said that women do not take credit for the work that they do, since being outgoing is something only men are familiar with. Over the last few years, there has been a drastic change in the way men and women think.

Tantric sex is a firm follower of the fact that men and women do have opposite characteristics. This is the elementary principle of the Tantra. The eastern theories claim that Yin represents feminism while Yang represents masculinity. But there is no concrete proof that a woman cannot have Yang characteristics or that a man cannot have Yin characteristics. Rather than viewing men and woman as two entities, you should begin to focus on the energies. The Tantra believes in the amalgamation of these two energies.

Shiva and Shakti

The most common image of the Yin and the Yang is the Hindu divine couple Lord Shiva and Goddess Shakti. Lord Shiva represents the entire universe since he is considered the creator and Goddess Shakti represents the root of all energy. The union of the two deities creates a longing in you and every other human being to be treated as a god or a goddess. This is discussed in detail in the following chapters. You will learn to worship your partner as a god or a goddess.

The male energy that is found in Lord Shiva represents ecstasy while the energy in Goddess Shakti represents wisdom. This magical combination is what helps a person attain enlightenment. This perfect couple is always represented in numerous entwined positions – either dancing, or embracing or standing together. There are other positions where Goddess Shakti is wrapped around Lord Shiva with her legs propped around his hips. The dancing position by far is the most sacred since they are able to free their spirit, giving them a chance to attain enlightenment.

Understanding the opposites

You may have made divisions amongst you and your partner. You have to first identify and understand these divisions to strike a balance between the opposite energies. There are quite a few stereotypical characteristics that you may relate to. You will have to identify those characteristics and make note of them. You have to go from one extreme to the next. You should ask your partner to do this too. You will then have to see how you can embrace the extreme characteristics that you and your partner have. You have to identify how you can strike a balance between the polarities that exist between you and your partner. You will have to identify the Yin to your partner's Yang and vice versa.

You might now wonder if it is true that opposites attract. Sit back and think for yourself. You will be able to answer this question on your own. Try analyzing your past relationships. See how you and your partner were different from each other. Identify whether the differences were complemented by each other. This will help you analyze your future relationships as well.

My partner is my beloved

Tantra is not mad love but sacred love. You are honoring your partner and cherishing your partner while making love. You will shower unconditional love on your partner. When you are talking to your partner, use loving words like 'darling' or 'beloved'. You will find that those little words have aroused feelings of love within your partner. Call your partner with the aforementioned loving words when talking about him or her in public. You might find it terribly strange to do so but you will be sending out a message of love to the person you are speaking to.

The Desire Spectrum

You will find yourself with new views of desire. You may feel a desire every time you think of someone. You may comment on how you want a guy or how hot a girl is when you see them passing. You only feel these desires when you feel incomplete. Since you feel incomplete, you always want another person. You find yourself feeling needy and feeling wanted. But when you do get the person you want, you begin to want something more. You want someone prettier, more interesting and sometimes someone richer. Through tantric sex, you will be able to detach yourself from superficial needs. This will help you create a healthier relationship with your partner.

You feel empowered to say what you want!
When you find yourself empowered, you are able to set boundaries both during sex and in life in general. You find yourself with a new level of self – esteem. In tantric sex, you OWN your body and your soul. When your partner wants you to enter you, he must ask for your permission. You should not be afraid and have to say yes or no as the situation demands. You have to stop and say that you do not want to be touched in a way that is not comfortable with. You empower your partner when you speak the truth this way. You will be giving your partner the methods to use to please you. You have to be okay with how you are touched and how you feel.

Chapter 13 Teachings of tantric sex

In this chapter we will look at certain teachings of tantra that will help you increase the intimacy; sexual pleasure and it will also help you change your life and relationships for the better. When these teachings are made proper use of then they can also help you take a step closer to enlightenment. Each one of these teachings can be used in two ways, a sexual and a non-sexual way.

Breathe

Remember to breathe. If you have noticed, then you would have realized that a lot of importance has been given to breathing in almost all the teachings that have originated in the East and these teachings can help you attain enlightenment. It is essential that you understand why this is done and the manner in which it is related to Tantra and spiritual development as well.

The answer is quite simple, we all breathe all the time and if we stop breathing for too long it might result in death or becoming unconscious. In this manner, it can be understood that breath is related to our consciousness. Breath can be thought of as energy; every breath we take fills our body with a fresh burst of oxygen and takes away the carbon dioxide. This oxygen is in turn supplied to all the cells in the body. Breath and oxygen can be thought of as fundamental needs of our body. Breathing is not a conscious but an unconscious function. You might not pay attention to whether or not you are breathing, but you never really stop breathing till the day you die. Your life is dependent on something that you don't even do voluntarily.

What would happen if we were to make breathing a conscious effort? All the teachings from the East, including Tantra, make relating a conscious function and this will help transform the way the practitioner of these functions. Like I have stated earlier, breath is energy. And by being able to regulate your breathing, you will be able to regulate the energy generated as well.

You might be able to notice some interesting things if you can focus on not just your own breathing, but also that of your partner while engaged in a sexual activity. It is quite common that while having sex, people engaged in it tend to either hold in their breath for a few moments when they get excited. And then they let out a lot of the air that they were holding on to. When you halt your breathing in such a manner and then let it all out by a jolt, then the energy flowing in your body is likely to be disrupted as well. When you make breathing a conscious act during sex, you will learn how to control the movement of energy instead of just allowing it to flow in the body.

This teaching of tantra is all about breathing in a relaxed manner, take deep breaths, do not stop breathing and don't tighten your lungs. Let the breath flow freely. Only when you do this will the energy flow through your body freely. When your breathing is short or even shallow, this ends up choking the energy in our body.

If you want to achieve a full-body orgasm then it becomes easy when you breathe deeply. Focus on your breathing and allow it to move without any restrictions in your body. Feel the breath filling and then leaving your lungs fully.

Relax

In the same manner, in which shallow breathing can obstruct the flow of energy while participating in sex, the tension in your muscles will also do the same. The muscular tension that you experience during sexual activity is not a conscious one, but an unconscious one. The principle of tantric sex is to make this muscular tension a conscious decision to help you become aware of all the muscles that are being held up. You do require some tension to facilitate the movement if body and for also holding up the body, but that's about it. Muscular tension is not needed everywhere.

If you make the decision of tensing up your muscles a conscious one, you will observe that during sex you tend to tense up some muscles unnecessarily. A man might tense up his muscles even while enjoying oral sex. All he needs to do is lie down on his back and enjoy the ministrations provided to him by his partner; even then he might end up tensing his muscles in his torso and legs. In this case, you would notice that none of this tension is required. Let the energy flow without any restrictions in the body. Focus your attention on not just relaxing your muscles but also on breathing. Enjoy the warmth of the sexual energy that is flowing through your body.

However, it is essential that you understand that relaxation is required of not just your body but your mind as well. Let go of all the expectations, just enjoy the activities you are involved in. bask in the warmth of this energy. Let go of all the unnecessary emotions; don't hold yourself back.

Sounds can help!

Sounds are critical for the movement of energy as well. Some people might not be comfortable or they might even be self-conscious or nervous about the way they sound, but don't take this consideration seriously while considering tantric sex.

Let go of all your inhibitions. Express yourself freely and without any restrictions. Make all those sounds that can express the way you are feeling while engaged in the act. These sounds that you make involuntarily can be referred to as connected sounds. That is, these sounds are connected with the emotions or even sensations that you are experiencing. These sounds will help in the unobstructed flow of energy in your body.

If you are quiet or silent, then the movement of energy becomes difficult. But when you are loud or vocal, then the energy can start moving freely in your body. The more sounds you make, the pleasure quotient you experience will also be more. So, the noise you make is directly proportional to the pleasure you experience. The more connected these sounds are to your emotions and sensations, the more freely and powerfully the energy can move within your body.

If you trying to decipher the sounds associated with each of these emotions and come up blank, don't worry, because these sounds will be generated only while you are experiencing something. Think about all the pleasurable times, it might make you gasp or moan slightly, some experiences might just cause you to intake a sharp breath. All these will contribute to the sounds that you make while engaged in sexual intercourse. Everything that you feel has a sound. The sound produced need not be coherent, it is just about expressing your emotions in a vocal manner.

While having sex, there might be some experiences that make you feel ecstatic and this will be expressed in the sounds you make. But on the other hand, there might be some experiences that might be unpleasant or painful. Do not hold back on these sensations, if something seems painful, and then make the sound that you are in pain. This will help in letting your partner know that you are in pain. It is not just about being vocal, but you can be verbal as well. Verbal means making use of words to express what you are feeling whereas vocal means the making use of sounds to communicate the same. You have the liberty to say what you are feeling, if you feel that something is unpleasant or painful, express it. If you feel that something is pleasurable or just perfect express that as well. Do not hold back your emotions. When you express yourself through sounds, the energy tends to move faster than while expressing through words.

You can consider the example of a toddler who has just acquired speech. At this age, they communicate their feelings through the sounds they make. Think about a child throwing a tantrum, the gamut of angry sounds they make can help the parent understand that the child is cranky and requires something. All you hear would be a jumble of sounds and hardly any words. Even if words were present, the words would be to the point like a loud "No". Toddlers are capable of expressing their emotions loudly, whether be it their laughter or the wails of their sadness. This is how they express their emotions.

And in the same manner, let go of your inhibitions. Make sounds that you want to, it doesn't matter what they sound like either to you or your partner, because these sounds are capable of expressing what you are experiencing at a particular moment. The more you keep doing this, the deeper and connected your sexual activity will be and the result will also be much better.

It is really important that I stress the importance of this point. Of all the principles of tantra, this seems to be the one that a lot of people struggle with. Let go of your inhibitions and express yourself freely.

Eye contact is essential

This might sound pretty basic and obvious to some extent. But it really does help make your sexual experience more pleasurable, enjoyable and intense. Looking at your partner while engaged in any sexual act will definitely make the experience more intense. When I say eye contact, I don't mean that you should stare wistfully into the eyes of your partner. Move over the longing look a love-struck puppy has in its eyes, we are talking about some serious X-rated gazing, so get ready for it. This way will definitely help you attain some extra intimacy. For getting started you and your partner can find a comfortable spot to sit so that you both will be able to look into each other's eyes. Take a moment to gather your concentration; usually, a deep breath will do the trick. Once you feel that you are ready, you can open your eyes and gaze into those of your partner. Allow your partner the access to see you, your true self, and in the same manner, you can gaze at them. This might feel a little stupid initially, but trust me when I say that this little trick is extremely effective. And this trick provides you the liberty to incorporate it whenever you want to.

Allow yourself to communicate through your eyes and not just your genitals. You can let your eyes wander over each other's body. Let your partner see the lust in your eyes and the wanton abandonment. Nothing would be a better turn on than knowing that your partner desires you and needs you. In the manner that sounds and touch can communicate, in the same way, you can communicate a lot more by making use of just your eyes alone. This will help you both communicate with each other in an earnest manner.

Pay attention

Energy flows where the attention goes, is a popular saying in the tantric circles. You will have to concentrate on how and where you want the energy to flow. If you are looking to achieve a full-body orgasm, then you will need to focus on your entire body. You will have to pay some attention to feeling those highly sexualized feelings in all your cells as well. A woman who wants to achieve a splendid vaginal orgasm will have to concentrate her attention to deep within herself and pry out all the sexual sensations hiding within. You can make use of the breathing technique and also of muscle relaxation, as well as eye contact coupled with sound to focus your attention and draw out your energy to the spot where you want it to go to. You can choose to focus only on your genitals the place where the sexual energy is stored.

The philosophy of tantra suggests that an individual should let the sexual energy spread all through the body instead of confining it to just one area. To facilitate the energy to move from the genitals and spread through all the different cells. This energy can be used to help revitalize the body or for any other sexual purpose. The energy flow will be where your attention is. So concentrate on that while engaging in sex.

Always be present

The underlying principle of all the teachings is to be present. Present does not just imply being physically present, but mentally present as well. Be present in the moment. Do not wander off to your dreamland or fantasize about anything else. Try to be in the moment with your partner. Be present in what is happening.

Often it so happens that people end up zoning off to their fantasy world while engaged in sex. They close their eyes and drift to their fantasy realms instead of being present in the lovemaking. Sometimes men also do this on purpose. They can think about something completely non sexual to postpone their ejaculation. This is thought of as being unnecessary in tantra or anything associated to energy work. If you are present, you will be able to endure more of what is happening around you. Only when you are fully aware of what is happening around you will you be able to experience the moment to the fullest. Energy goes where the attention does, and if your attention is fixated on something entirely different, then even your energy will follow suit. Focus your energy on yourself and your lover. Try to be in the moment; do not lose focus of that. And when this happens the potential of seeking greater pleasure will be diminished.

These principles will surely help you to have a better sexual experience when implemented.

Chapter 14 Understand the Challenges Created by Social Messages

These social messages and myths create an array of challenges in both women's and men's sexuality and inhibit people's ability to form satisfying and fulfilling sexual and emotional connections. As a result of these harmful myths and damaging social messages, many relationships end up full of misunderstanding, hurt, and resentment. Instead of seeing these differences and the problems they cause as a result of socialization, people often take them personally or judge their partner inadequate. These differences have negative outcomes for women, men, and couples, and they lead to low sexual desire and dysfunction for women, midlife crisis and dysfunction for men, sexless or low-sex relationships, and emotional disconnection.

Challenges for Women

Distractibility During Sex
Social messages cause women to be distanced from their sexuality and much more easily distracted from their sexual feelings than men are.

They are worried about whether or not it is okay to have sex or are self-conscious about their bodies. Thus it becomes easy for little interruptions to cause women's arousal to drop suddenly. Intrusive thoughts about responsibilities can come in and ruin the mood as well.

Loss of Sexual Interest as a Mom

The image of a good mother is that she is pure, giving, and sexless. Women are supposed to live up to the social ideal of being a perfect caregiver, focused completely on her children. This image makes mothers feel like their needs are selfish, that sex or any other sensual, self-caring pursuits should be suppressed. We've heard so many women say that, when they became mothers, they didn't feel right doing all of the "naughty" sexual activities they once did. They stopped having many of the experiences that used to make them most aroused.

Low Sexual Desire

Many people try to figure out if women's lower desire is socially or biologically determined; we believe it is likely a bit of both. Because of hormonal differences, women have a somewhat lower sex drive; however, as we have explained, social messages also make it hard for women to connect to their sexual selves and cultivate their desire. Women have very high and usually unattained potential for pleasure: they generally experience more full-body sensation than men and can have varied and multiple orgasms. If your partnership has a woman in it, we want to help you move beyond the harmful social messages so that she can experience her full erotic potential.

Challenges for Men

Midlife Crisis

Social messages are often what lead to men's midlife crisis. When we think of midlife crisis, what often comes to mind is a fortysomething man in a shiny red hot rod running off with some younger woman to find himself. Popular representations of this phenomenon paint this man as childish and selfish. The movie fantasy is generally that he wises up, realizes the error of his ways, repents, and returns to his wife and family. This popular depiction misses the point in many ways: it fails to address the underlying emotional, physiological, and societal reasons for this phenomenon. Men's bodies experience an abrupt and significant change in ability near age forty. As men are noticing their own physical decline, many are also seeing their fathers get old or die, which leads them to wonder whether they will get to live their lives the way they want to before they themselves die. The definitions of "good husband" and "good father" rarely leave space for men to continue doing the things they love to do in life without being deemed selfish and uncaring.

Sexual Dysfunction

Men may experience a psychological shutdown to sex because it feels terrible that their partner keeps rejecting their sexual advances. They don't want to push their sexual desires on their partner and are tired of feeling rejected so they stop getting erections. In addition, there is so much pressure on men to be sexual and ready for every sexual invitation that they aren't allowed the build-up they need to stay connected to their partner during sex. Instead, they worry about their performance. Many men experience anxiety and performance issues such as erectile dysfunction, early ejaculation, and delayed ejaculation. In these cases, we think sexual dysfunction is a response to a dysfunctional situation. If a man feels rejected or pushed to perform on command, his penis begins to rebel, as if to say, "I don't like this treatment" or "You can't make me do that." The fact that his penis is saying "no" to things that he doesn't want means it's time to take a look at the situation and see if there is something that needs to change in the relationship, not in him.

Challenges for Couples

Sexless Relationship/Marriage

Many couples come to us because they find themselves in sexless marriages. These marriages might be wonderful in every other way, with plenty of love, companionship, commitment, and cooperation, but one or both partners feel no sexual attraction or desire for the other. This can be a result of the different social messages they received. Sexless marriage can also be a result of partners having different desires (see "Hottest Sexual Movies" below) and not knowing how to communicate the differences. It may also simply be that one or both of them has lost attraction for the other.

As a result of social messages, women experience low desire and men feel inadequate and overwhelmed with sexual urges. This is not always the case, as a man can be very repressed around his sexuality and his partner more open due to an accepting sexual socialization. In general, however, the one who wants sex more will try to initiate and get rebuffed repeatedly. Eventually, that person will begin to feel rejected and undesirable, give up, and stop trying.

There is nothing inherently wrong with having a sexless marriage, provided that you are honest with each other and agree that it is what you want. If either or both of you want sex, then you may be able to learn how to reconnect with each other sexually. This section will help you find the energy, playfulness, and technique to meet each other's sexual needs. Alternatively, you may have to face your disappointment about your loss of desire and attraction and figure out how you will handle it. Reading about disappointment in Part 2 of this book can be helpful.

Emotional Distance

Men's and women's differing socialization can lead to a relationship that lacks intimacy, empathy, and connection. It is much easier to have empathy for someone when you can understand and relate to their feelings, fears, and desires. Because women's sexuality is repressed and men's emotionality is repressed, relationships can be full of emotional misunderstanding. In relationships, women often feel overly emotional or "too much," and men get labeled as emotionally unavailable. Because they are repressed and their expression is usually less overt, men's emotions can end up being left out.

Affairs

The emotional distance and sexless relationships that result from all of this misunderstanding often lead to affairs. One partner feels like some of their deep sexual or emotional needs are not being fulfilled. Often they still love their partner and try to get those needs met elsewhere without breaking up their relationship or family.

One Couple's Plight Through the Lens of Social Messages

Mandy and Phillip came to us seven years into their marriage. Phillip dragged Mandy into the session because he wanted to have a better sexual connection with her. He shared that he had felt so much closer to Mandy when they had an active sex life, and he missed their connection. Mandy had not wanted to come because she thought sex was the only thing Phillip wanted from her. She also said that sex was not pleasurable and was sometimes painful for her. She felt like Phillip just wanted to use her and that he didn't care about her or their children. They both had very time-consuming careers, and Mandy felt that any spare time they had should be focused on their co-parenting. Phillip felt that they both gave a lot of time and energy to being parents, and he missed the wild woman he'd married.

They spoke of each other in very judgmental terms. Phillip described Mandy as "frigid," while Mandy said Phillip had a "one-track mind" and didn't care about anything but sex. Mandy did not want Phillip to touch her in any way, because she was suspicious that any time Phillip tried to physically connect with her it was only because he was trying to get sex. They spent the entire session blaming and shaming each other for how they'd ended up, which was so clearly shaped by the social messages they'd been given.

It took them three years to come back for a second session, and by then they were on the verge of divorce. Mandy had caught Phillip cheating, and they were both overwrought. Phillip shared, "I tried everything to get Mandy to see that I was invested in our family and the children, but I just started to feel like I was dead inside, like there was nothing left that made me want to get out of bed anymore. I couldn't even get it up to masturbate." Mandy added, "I didn't realize how depressed Phillip was, but I can't believe he went outside the marriage and betrayed me like that! I still can't believe that sex is more important than anything else to him, even his family."

It took Mandy and Phillip months to begin to see how badly they had missed and misunderstood each other. Because Mandy had been taught that sex was dirty and unimportant, she didn't realize it was one of the main ways that Phillip felt accepted and emotionally connected to her. Phillip realized that he had been judging Mandy harshly, calling her frigid without realizing how she was struggling to be herself in the midst of the pressure to be a good girl, a good wife, and a good co-worker. As they started to see that they were both longing for deep connection as well as self-expression, they began to support each other and forgive each other for all the misperceptions and judgments. We were sorry to see that it had to get to this point of devastation before they were willing to really face each other's needs and feelings.

Chapter 15 Romance After The Kids

Children are wonderful little human beings, and as your family grows, you will most often find that your relationship with your spouse can suffer. It's not the fault of the kids though. They just happen to take up a lot of your time, and life as you knew it is changed. Now, whenever you want to go somewhere you have to plan ahead, so any spontaneity that you once enjoyed with your spouse has been thrown out the window. Children create more mess; therefore your daily chores multiply significantly. They are also very demanding of your attention, so you end up spending less time with your husband or wife, and have what seems to be no time to yourself at all. But, having children doesn't mean that the romance has to die between couples. You just need to have a plan in action to ensure you still get the time you need to have some adult time.

Update Each Other Every Week

Parents can often feel like passing ships – one is often running out the door just as one is running in. With work schedules and kids to take care of, there's little time to go round. This is particularly true when your children are very young, as they have no independence skills, so they have to rely on their parents entirely. A trap couples often fall into is one of moaning about the negatives that have taken place during the week. To prevent this from happening, set aside some time (even if it's just half an hour) each week where you and your spouse can sit down and update each other about the week that has just passed. Make an effort to share something positive that has happened, or a funny story about something the kids have done that the other might not be aware of. Then, talk about a negative event that occurred. Try and keep the positive and negative comments even, so if you have 3 positives, only talk about 3 negatives. This little bit of time you share with each other every week can make a lot of difference towards keeping up communication between you. It will also help you reconnect with your spouse after such a hectic week.

Sharing the Parenting

Sometimes, depending on work requirements, one parent may feel that they are taking on the full job of taking care of the kids and the house. Try and create a schedule so both parents are involved in the childcare, and both have some time out. Having time to destress can change your mood and how you interact with your spouse and your children, and this makes for a happier household. When the burden of raising children is shared, even if it's not entirely equal, both parents will feel as though they are cooperating with each other and working together. The reason this can enhance the romance in your marriage is because if you are both more relaxed, and one doesn't feel as though they are doing more than the other, then you both will feel supported and appreciate your partner more.

Finding Time for Intimacy

Finding the time to be intimate with your spouse can be extremely difficult, especially when the children are babies or toddlers. Half of them won't sleep during the night, so you may be up and down all night settling your child. It's very hard to relax and feel romantic if you constantly have one ear out listening for the sounds of a crying baby. Then, of course, there is the exhaustion, especially during the baby years. Raising and taking care of a baby takes a lot of energy, and in this modern world, many mothers have to return to work early on to help support the family. So, you have work during the day, chores at night, and child-caring duties to take care of before you can even think about slipping into bed. Then you can almost guarantee that as soon as you start something in the bedroom, the little one will have a screaming fit, or a nightmare. Wait till they're older and they burst into the room unannounced! It's no wonder that intimacy and romance often falls to the wayside once children come along. So how on earth do you find the time? Well, it's definitely no easy task, but with a bit of planning and by becoming opportunists, it can be done. In the first instance, send baby to grandma's for the night. A night to yourselves can be hugely rewarding. If that's not possible, then you need to be ready for any opportunity that may arise. If your baby is in the early phases of sleep, take the chance. If your baby wakes up and you are in the middle of an intimate moment, remember that it doesn't hurt to let them cry for a few minutes. Learn to switch off temporarily from the crying sounds. This isn't easy for many people, especially mothers, but it can become a necessity. You need to find time for intimacy on a regular basis, or you may end up in a relationship where intimacy has completely gone.

Get Yourselves a Babysitter

For any chance at romance after children, you need to find yourselves a really good babysitter that you can trust. This could be a relative that takes your child for the night or someone who comes into your home and watches your child for you. If you have to hire a babysitter it may cost you a little money, but the time you get to spend alone with each other will be well worth it. Get out of the house, away from all the chaos, and just enjoy spending time with your spouse. Don't be tempted to ring the babysitter every 5 minutes to check up on them either. If you hire someone you trust, you have nothing to worry about. Make sure you hire them for more than an hour or two as well. It will take you a while to wind down and relax, so there's no point going out for an hour then coming back.

For some couples, it is more helpful if they book a night at a motel or hotel. Completely getting away can really help couples relax and get in the mood for romance and intimacy. Far better than being at home surrounded by laundry, dishes, toys, and diapers.

Pay More Attention To Your Spouse

When they are little, and in some cases when they are older, children have no manners when it comes to interrupting adults. You may be on the phone and have a toddler pulling on your sleeve the whole time demanding your undivided attention. Or as a couple, you may be having a conversation and all you can hear next to you is mum…mum…mum…This is extremely frustrating, for the mother that is being harassed and the father that is trying to have a conversation. At first, this will seem very difficult to do, but you must learn how to ignore your child. Temporarily of course! Children are very distracting and your concentration levels drop significantly when being interrupted, so the sooner you can teach them not to do it the better. If the child absolutely demands your attention right now and you can't even listen to your spouse, then explain to your spouse that you will just sort the child out then get straight back to the conversation. As your child gets a little older, there are other things you can do to prevent interruptions. If as a couple you like to spend time after dinner talking over coffee or a glass of wine, explain to the child that every night after dinner they are to go and play for 30 minutes. Tell them you will come and get them when the time is up, or give them an electronic timer so they can see the minutes ticking down. This half an hour gives you the opportunity to talk to each other and reconnect.

Appreciation, Admiration and Affection

These three words are ones you need to ingrain in your mind for future reference. No matter how busy or how bad a day you have had, remember to show each other some appreciation, admiration and affection. Tell your spouse how you appreciate the help they have given you that day, or because they have stepped in and taken over one of the chores when they got home. Let your partner know you admire how they handled a particular situation involving the children. It could be for dealing with a sick child, or having to reprimand the child. And always show your partner some form of affection every single day. It could be a gentle touch, a kiss, a love note, or telling your partner they look nice today. Every person is looking for these 3 things from someone; it's what we all crave. Someone to show that they care and that they are thankful for our support. Making your spouse feel worthwhile will increase their self-esteem, and romance will be rekindled.

Chapter 16 Improving Intimacy

People often express their desire to love and be loved, to be accepted and known for who we are, to be in a safe relationship, hoping to share out failings and dreams. Is it intimacy that people truly want?

There are so many times when people will use the term intimate in a completely physical context. People can call a couple intimate to express the fact that they have a sexual relationship. But the truth is that this is a narrow and misleading use of the word because there are different types of intimacy:

- Emotional
- Sexual
- Experiential
- Intellectual

Sexual Intimacy

There are times when everybody hungers for a sexual connection, and this is a physical longing. We may not only yearn for intercourse, but also just the presence and touch of another person with their own sensual splendor; the textures, sounds, scents, tastes, and the visual aspects also play a part.

During sex, barriers are lowered, and another person is allowed to your private personal space. This type of intimacy involves some trust and vulnerability. There will be times when everybody wants sex and not lovemaking. This can happen without any attachments, with a bit of affection, or between friends. If you pay attention, you can understand the little nuances of sharing your body and not your heart.

Emotional Intimacy

Sometimes we are interested in finding an emotional connection; accepting yourself, loving yourself, sharing happiness and tough times. People crave comfort, closeness, and trust. People want to have a special connection with a person on a deep emotional level.

This type of intimacy doesn't need physical affection, though for some it can be enhanced by holding hands or a kiss on the cheek.

Two people can be married for years, and they never reach emotional intimacy; remember that intimacy is not a destination but an experience or a group of feelings. Communication is important when it comes to emotional intimacy, but people tend to communicate about life superficially.

People also use activities, humor, and sarcasm to fill up the time they spend together. Whether intentional or not, people tend to "deflect and protect" so that they can avoid transparency and vulnerability that people need in order to thrive as a couple.

The vulnerability that is needed for emotional intimacy produces anxiety for many people. A good way to help get rid of this anxiety is to allow plenty of time to pass so that you can establish trust. The vulnerability can still prove to be tough especially if you're out of practice.

While many people view sex as a relationship glue from where intimacy and communication will flow, others see emotional intimacy as a prerequisite to a good sex life. So, what if this vulnerability isn't going to happen? What if your significant other isn't willing, or can't communicate on a deep and personal way? Even if you have amazing sex, will an unsatisfying amount of emotional intimacy leave you wanting more?

Everybody Experiences Intimacy Differently

Sexual and emotional intimacy tends to be tricky because there are no absolutes. What everybody needs when it comes to intimacy can vary. The way one person deeply shares will be different than the next.

In the same way, our comfort with emotional and sexual intimacy is going to change some over time and evolve with the relationship we're in and the circumstances. Take this, for example, a woman who was married for 20 years is now divorced. To say the very least, the mere thought of stripping off in front of a new lover may cause anxiety, so she could choose to establish a mutual emotional intimacy foundation before any sexual activity. Or she could go the route of detachment with a hookup instead of putting her heart out there.

There are some people that are found with keeping sex at arm's length from their emotions, which makes their lives a lot less complicated. There are single mothers out there that explicitly operate like this, given that having to deal with their ex, raising their kids, and hold down a job is an emotional overload.

There are others that need a convergence of sexuality with connection, agreement, transparency, and trust, which is the definition of emotional intimacy. This all depends on communication and time.

But passion isn't decided through emotional intimacy, just like emotional intimacy doesn't have to have any physical contact. Love is able to happen at an emotional remove or even a sexual remove for that matter. Connection, sex, love: these are what make up the best mix of satisfaction and comfortableness for both people in a relationship.

How to Deepen Your Sexual Connection

If you're interested in bringing more intimacy into your sex life with your partner, instead of it just being sex, here are five things that can help deepen that intimacy.

> 1. Realize the importance of creating an intimate friendship with your significant other

A lot of people tend to focus too much on the technique during sex. However, your relationship with your partner is a lot more important for feelings of intimacy. The sense of safety, mutual trust, and emotional connection in your relationship is needed in order to bring the intimacy to your sexual desires. Basically, you should work up to the feeling that you are living with somebody that you crave so much, that makes the actual sex even more pleasurable.

2. Become deeply connected with your body
All the stresses of every day like can keep many of us from being able to keep a thorough and consistent self-care routine. As a result, many will devote only a small amount of time enjoying, embracing, and exploring our own bodies. The effects of stress will often trickle into the sex life. When a person doesn't have an intimate and comfortable relationship with their self, it's almost impossible to create an intimate and comfortable sexual relationship with their partner. If you make a space to love, feel, and explore your own body, you will be able to communicate better about what you want, what makes you feel fulfilled, and what you crave.

3. Speak up

A big reason as to why sex will begin to feel like a routine, and a lot less passionate, is because there isn't enough communication. You may see it as overreacting if you voice how upset you were when your partner gave your friend flirty eyes. It would seem unnecessary to speak about how upset you were when your partner didn't ask your opinion when planning your date. But look at it this way: when you suppress your emotion, it isn't going to go away, it will show up again somewhere else.

A way that it will show up is through suppressed intimacy, any form of intimacy. If you can shorten the time between when you were upset about letting that person know, the lower your resentment levels will be. Less negativity means you will have a better willingness to receive and give in different ways, especially with sex.

4. *Embrace the dark, light, and everything in between*

It's easy for couples to fall into sexual monotony, and it typically coexists with safety. But if you can widen your expressiveness range, it can open the door to a deeper spiritual connection, and this typically means getting out of your safety zone. You may be worried about bringing up something that is "bad," but stepping into that area could be what you need. During sex, it could mean letting your partner take you with more abandon and strength.

5. Surrender to what happens

A lot of the disconnection during sex can come from the pressure of achieving something. This could mean having an orgasm, trying to look good, or being seen as good in bed. It will distract you from the beauty and sacredness of the moment. Maybe you should look at the outcome as experiencing this moment with your partner. If you weren't pressured into reaching a milestone while being intimate, how deeper could your relationship go, and surrender to your partner?

Chapter 17 More Intimacy in 7 Days

You just have to mesmerize your partner with mind-blowing sex to really keep them and have deep bonding with them. Just a quickie in the bathtub or some dry kisses before rolling over will not cut it. You need to satisfy your partner in some well-planned steamy sex session that will leave them always horny anytime they are around you, in fact, they can't literally get their hands off you. Having a bomb ass sex with your partner will make you the woman feeling sexier while the man will have a deep connection with you. it is good to make sex a lot more fun that will drive your partner crazy, use sultry sex positions that will make them explode in ecstasy and will help remind him or her always why you are in a relationship with your them

It is pertinent you turn to sex positions that will strengthen or build the deep connection you need with your partner. .whether you are trying to rekindle the flames of a real love or trying to foster a more profound link with someone new, you need to try out the below hot sex positions that will enable you both to always be in the mood for intense orgasmic sex session filled with fire and deep connection. This will aid your partner fall in love with you all over again.

- Side by side position

You can get your love flames burning very high for deep connection using this sex position. This sex position will leave you both gasping for breathe after the hot sex session and it will foster deep connection because of eye contact and physical closeness it afford the partners during the sex session. With this sizzling position, you and your partner will be delving into a new world of pleasure because the position offers the man the opportunity to get explicit access to your woman's G-spot while pleasuring himself too. This position also promotes deep bonding and makes the woman sexier through the eyes gazing by the partners, kissing is done effortlessly, and there is ease of communication too since the partners can see one another's responses to stimulation. This sex position begins with the man and woman lying side by side by each other; the man draped his leg over the woman's hip so that he can pull the woman's vagina deeper into him. The woman can sometimes have her knees bent up to her breasts for a deeper penetration. To heighten the sexual heat the man should ask the woman to part her thigh a bit, the man would then use his cock to rub her clitoris and allow her scream in excitement for a while before penetrating deeply and thrusting forth and back again still both climax.

- Spooning position

This is a perfect sex position that will make partners scream off their lungs in ecstasy as the pleasure one another, this position is both a sexual position and a cuddling technique, so one can imagine the orgasmic thrills partners will enjoy when using this hot sex position. This sex position will leave the woman feeling sexier and having a strong connection with her partner. The position is a rear-entry position which is like the doggy style position and it is ideal for partners that need a deeper and more pleasurable sensation, it a great position since it allows partners to work through the action of sex together. Spooning sex position puts less strain on the muscles which makes the couple last for long while making love. This sex position has the man lying on his side while the woman lies in front of the man facing away, so this means that the woman will be in the inner spoon position while the man will be in the outer spoon position preparing for the entry penetration. The man enters her from behind; the man can add more sensation by grabbing and fondling with her breast from behind, stimulating her clitoris and finally going anal with her before climaxing.

- Doggy style

A psychosexual therapist based in Palo Alto, California, said that this sex position gives partners orgasmic thrills especially the women deep penetration that leads to immense pleasure and can help the partner have some deep connection after the steamy sex session. So if you need a sex position that will give your partner the adrenaline rush and keep sexual flames burning in the relationship while also keeping you the woman sexier and create deep connection for you both in the relationship, then using the doggy style will just be it. The doggy sex position is pretty easy the woman lies on her stomach with her butt in the air, maybe with a pillow under her pelvis for extra support, the man stands behind her to penetrate from behind but before then he can stimulate the clitoris to bliss with a vibrator. The man can make the woman scream more by introducing anal sex and cap it up with vagina sex but must apply plenty of lube and continue deep thrusting still the both erupt in multiple orgasms.

- The chair sex position

You can't get it wrong with this naughty sex position especially when it comes to sex making that will create deep bonding because of the close body contact involved with this position. The position gets the man all excited since he will be the one sitting and taking in all erotic view of the entire woman's body. The woman on the other hand who is on top of the man will be having it easier with the stimulation of her clitoral and G-spot with this position. The good thing about this position is that it enables the partners to find the right spots to stimulate and the intensity and speed can build up from there. The position will help the partners ditch the bed for a chair so using the chair than a bed will add some zing to the already sizzling sex position. So you can check out the chair position because it will not only add romp to your sex session but foster deep connection and intimacy with your partner. This sex position start with the man sitting upright on the chair and the woman sitting on the man but backing him, The man can start with foreplay like fondling, fingering and stimulating the clitoris and massaging each other bodies, then the woman gently now direct the erect cock to her vagina and lean forward so that she can have the ease of deep penetration while moving her hips up and down in circles which could be backward or forward. To heighten the sexual pleasure the woman can turn around to stimulate all the erogenous zones with her hands and mouth and this will help put fire on both bodies, drawing you both together to create a better connection that can't be denied. The man can take over now and ride the woman to stupor with some deep thrusting.

- Woman on top sex position

Woman on top sex position is a build up on the missionary sex position where the woman is on top. This sex position is classic for partners that really want to connect emotionally with one another through good sex. Apart from the hot sex romp, this sex position offers partners it also offers deep connection through direct eye contact, sexy sounds and sensual touches and there is much more control of deep penetration too with this sex position. This sex position according to Zoldbrod will help the woman on top have clitoral stimulation which will make her reach multiple orgasms in the course of the sex session. This sex position can be started with the man lying on his back while the woman is comfortably on top, the woman grabs the man's penis and give it a huge blowjob to stretch the erection and to build up sensation before directing it to her vagina to insert, the woman leans her body forward and her hand beside or on the man head on the bed for support. The woman will then use her hips to rock back and forth or side by side till she can find the angle that let her rub her clitoris against the man's lower abdomen or pubic bone. This will make the man be practically caged inside the woman as she brings herself almost to climax. She can also engage the man's view by throwing her booty in his face while riding him hard forth and back. The man can be spanking the woman butt and responding to the rhythm of the ride still both climax.

- The lotus sex position

The lotus sex position is called the deep connection sex position because it provides face to face intimacy that can boost deep connection with a partner while making love. This sex position elicit excitement and erotic feelings, with this sex position the bodies are touching entirely and the partner's faces are close enough to have some fun together, there's intense eye contact, whispers, naughty talks and kisses are sure to follow with this sex position. If you need to feel sexier and have a deep connection with your partner then you need to try out the lotus sex position, you will sure have all that you had needed. Start this sex position with the woman sitting with her legs loosely crossed, while the man sits on top of the woman facing her and with his legs wrapped around the woman's back. The man penetrates the woman that way and focus now on moving up and down with slow sensual movement to build sexual thrills gradually. The woman can as well be grinding and rocking to the man rhythm, to build more orgasmic sensation the woman should put her arms under the man's arm and reach to grab his shoulders; this will make room for the woman to pull herself up and down on the man while intensely grinding and rocking him. There should be intermittent kissing, smooching, fondling, naughty talks etc in between. The man can heighten the pleasure to achieve back-arching, toe-curling screaming orgasm by thrusting and grinding deeply.

- Hold me sex position

Hold me a sex position can give partner spine-tingling pleasure while facilitating emotional intimacy and deep connection. This sex position will always leave the partner asking for more as the pleasure one another and also help to build the deepest connection because this sex position offers the opportunity of partners having eye contact, caressing and kissing themselves during the course of this sensational sex session. Hold me a sex position can be done anywhere so you can skip the bedroom and your usual routine with this sex position. This sex position will need the man standing upright and the woman first going on her knees to give the man a good suck on his cock, then she now jump on the man and the man need to hold the woman into his arms and the woman should wrap her legs around the man's waist and her arms should be around his neck. This is a typical sex position to promote body contact and connection as the partners come face to face with one another. Before penetrating the woman, the man can finger and stimulate her clit, kiss and suck away, then penetrate the woman now and grab her booty and push it forward so that he can have deep penetration. The woman can as well respond to the rhythm by pushing herself forth and back and to heighten the pleasure the man can place the woman's back against a wall for support and then thrust deeply till they both explode in multiple orgasms.

· Hands-**free sex position**

This is one sex position that apart from setting partners bodies on fire also connects them passionately when used. The outstanding feature of this sex position is that the sex position enables the partner's hands to be free for more arousal touches. Making love and have a good amount of fingering and erotic touches help ignite swirling sexual feelings and this can bring about massive excitement and thrills for the partners, such that a remembrance of lovemaking by the partner is fascinating and this will help keep them very close and deep into one another. This sex position promotes face to face contact for the partners which will enable them to smile at one another while also having very close eye contact too. Sex position of this nature can make partners be very emotional and want to always be in another arm. This sex has the man sit on a chair while the woman is astride facing him{ that is her legs wide apart on each side of the man's leg} and the woman's feet should be on the floor. This position will enable the man to face the woman, the same with the woman too. With them facing one another they can begin the lovemaking with foreplay, like the man giving the woman some tantalizing kisses, whispers into her ears, cuddle, fondle with the breast before penetrating. If the woman needs more intense pleasure she can be lifting her butt a bit higher while the man is thrusting and this can also help the man to have a deeper thrusting. The free hands they have because of this sex position can be used to rub, tingle and finger other erogenous spots of the body. The whole body feels thrilling sensation and the climax will be heavenly.

- Snow angel sex position

If you are looking for a smooth transition sex position away from your comfort sex style that will give mind-blowing orgasm, then this sex position will be perfect for you and your partner. This sex position would not only bring deep connections but will get your partner moaning and screaming in uncontrollable ecstasy. It is one sex position that hitting the G-spot is made easy and easily accessible as well as the man pleasuring himself to stupor. It just needs the woman to be flexible and agile to get this position right. This sex position has the woman lying on her back while the man is on top of her, the woman then draw her thighs into the man's chest and goes further to place her legs over her shoulders. This position will allow the man to bring the woman pelvis off the mattress, so that the tilt of the woman hips will allow the man to penetrate deeply into her with this position the man will have undeniable access to the woman G-spot. Rock the woman forth and back until the both climax with a bang.

- Missionary sex position

If you are looking for a sex position that will offer sexiness and deep connection in the bedroom then you should try out this good old sex position. No matter how old a trick maybe being creative with it will suffice. This is applicable too to this sex position you just have to use the creative angle that is written in this book. This sex position is perfect for boosting deep connection during lovemaking. From a personal view, this position allows the partners to be able to kiss, lock fingers together, and the proximity allows for some erotic talks that would arouse the partners even more. There is more connectedness with this position because partners will be wrapped in each other's arms, leg intertwined and a lot of eye contact and this will make the partners sexier, and lovemaking will be sweeter. This position can be called a man on top or couple facing each other. While the woman is on her back, the man climbs on top and penetrate the woman from there as in the right old fashioned way. You can add a rabbit vibrator to the mix to get the woman screaming and moaning away. The man can finger the woman's clitoris too to heighten the pleasure, then insert his penis again and thrust deeply until they both come in multiple orgasm.

Conclusion

By using the guidelines, we have set out in this book you can go on and experience the joys of an intimate, loving, sexual bond with your other half. Used correctly, these pointers are a powerful aid to achieving complete satisfaction.

By concentrating less on the amount of sex you are having and increasing the quality of sex, this can take pressure off couples. Ignore those annoying couples that are constantly banging on about "doing it" five times a week. That is not the path to satisfaction for everybody and you both need to agree that when you do have sex you are both in a place to make it great rather than concentrating on managing to have sex every other day!

Enjoy all your encounters! Orgasm or not, long hot sweaty session or a brief quickie before you set off for work. Sex between you should always create special memories and make you smile. Think about how you feel about your partner after sex, do you feel closer to them or do you detach completely afterward. Knowing how you should feel and how you actually feel may seem like a no brainer, but when was the last time you asked yourself how sex makes you feel?

Recognize when there is a lull in your sex life and know when to change things up! Follow some of the tips in this book and change your whole attitude to bedtime! Don't let modesty or embarrassment stop you experimenting with all manner of aids.

Be aware that other factors can affect your attitude to sex and learn how to address them. It is fairly obvious that the more care you show your body the more you will benefit from it when you are being intimate. A healthy body leads to healthy sex, right?? Mentally you also have to be in a good place to get the most out of your love life. If you are depressed or have other mental health issues then you need to seek treatment before you can concentrate on the physical side of your relationship.

Above all, if you are happy with your partner the sex will be better, simple, right? By using the tips to help you fall in love with your partner again you will glow with happiness and this will fuel your attraction to each other and lead to infinitely better sex!

MINDFULNESS SEX

Better sex to nurture love and to reach sexual health in the couple. How to build a relationship with awareness, mindful loving and sex. Sexual magic and magnetism power of love.

DONNA DARE

Description

Things are not always exactly the same, and marriage is not an exception. However, change is not always a bad thing. Even in the worst scenarios where you think things are going downhill or changing for worse, there is still an opportunity to turn them around. You must remember that everything has a solution, including even the worst scenarios. Most problems that you will face through marriage can be solved, but in order for this to happen, both parties need to be willing to try and do their best. Patience is the key. Don't expect things to work out in your first attempt. If they do, that's great, but if they don't, that's not a reason to stop. You need to keep trying until it works, no matter how many times you need to try. As with many other things, we have to try our best instead of giving up easily. It is only by giving the best of us that we can reach our goal and even when you have reached your goal, keep trying your best.

Marriage is a continuous process, so we need to try to be better at it every day. It is not enough with the "I do" you said a while ago; it is not enough with living together, having children or signing papers. In order to have a strong relationship, you need to continue to create positive experiences and a healthy environment. You need to keep working on your relationship, making each other feel good, important, desired, etc. There are so many ways to make your relationship stay alive and make each other feel special: a kiss, a touch, saying something nice, writing down a poem or message, doing something special for one another; those are things that are so easy to do and can be done often. Not everything has to be very elaborate and cost money. In fact, sometimes the smallest things can be the most meaningful. So, there are no excuses; no matter what gets in the way, there is always something we can do.

This guide will focus on the following:

- The psychology of sex
- Sex and spirituality
- Prepare mind and body for sex
- Keep your enemy closer
- Reconnect with your partner
- Breathing and diaphragmatic breathing
- Spin your chakras and breathe to ecstasy

- Develop sexual intuition
- Sexual massages
- Mindful oral sex
- Alternative sexual experiences... AND MORE!!!

Always look for different ways to help you and your partner work on your relationship.

Introduction

Romance stems from intimacy, as it is ultimately an extension of the intimacy itself. When there is intimacy in a relationship, you can be certain that some level of romance will prevail. If you want to have a really exciting sex life, you will want to build a solid foundation of intimacy and frost it off with a healthy helping of romance. Regardless of what someone's intimacy preference is, they will most certainly want to experience romance in their life. You can decide how you will display romance based on their preference for types of intimacy.

For Physical People

Anyone who likes physical intimacy will want to experience acts of romance in the physical sense. There are many ways that you can be romantic towards someone physically. When you are physically romantic, you want to do so with both sexual and non-sexual intentions. What that means is that while sometimes you are going to want to allow the romance to lead towards sex, you should not always allow for it to go that far. When you use physical intimacy to result in sex every single time, it can actually break down the value of this type of intimacy as your partner will begin to predict that every time you display physical romance, you want sex. You always want to keep your partner on edge and guessing. You can do this by mixing it up and sometimes going all the way and other times holding back and letting the passion build for a few days until you allow it to evolve into sexual romance.

Even if your partner likes physical romance, it doesn't mean they will like all physical touches. They may prefer some over others. Again, communication is the key to finding out what your partner likes. However, these are great places to start:

- Sensual massages
- Caressing or stroking
- Hugging
- Holding hands
- Cuddling or holding
- Kissing the face
- Kissing the lips

For Emotional People

For anyone who likes emotional intimacy, they will prefer acts of romance that stir up emotions inside of them. While physical touch will be one aspect of this, there are much more. In fact, in most cases, one of the other methods will be more likely to stir up the romance than physical touching will. Again, you want to use your actions as an opportunity to romance your partner whether you want to have sex or not. Especially with emotional people, using acts of romance only to have sex can lead to a greater sense of hurt feelings and it can actually heavily damage the intimacy between you and your partner, thus destroying the romance. If you want to succeed, you need to be willing to be romantic without sexual intentions on a regular basis, as well as romantic with sexual intentions from time to time.

If your partner likes emotional romance, you need to be certain that your romantic actions are always genuine. Those who are turned on by their emotions are often equally turned off by their emotions, and this can quickly destroy things in your relationship. Never commit an act of romance if it isn't genuinely coming from your heart. If you are, however, acting from your heart, the following ideas are a great place to start:

- Poetry
- Telling about how you feel
- Saying "I love you."
- Showing you care through words and actions
- Romantic gestures such as flowers or chocolate
- Remembering important things about them
- Looking into their eyes to establish an emotional connection

Stirring up the romance in your relationship is important if you want to have a strong sex life. Before you start focusing on new sex positions and how to spice up sex itself, you want to build a strong foundation. A relationship that is strong with intimacy and romance is one where sex will be uninhibited and much more enjoyable for both parties. It is important that you put in the groundwork to ensure that your relationship is strong outside of sex if you want to have mind-blowing sex that is incredible every single time.

In order to strengthen our marriage, we need balance; a balance in our sexual, romantic and physical connection. All of these things are important and they are connected one way or the other. So, if one is being affected, the others can eventually struggle as well. Don't believe that as time passes, we don't need to keep trying to please our partners; our needs will always remain the same. So instead of forgetting about these 3 aspects, we need to often nourish them. For couples who have a healthy relationship, it doesn't matter how long they have been together, they still enjoy each other's company and every day still feel like an adventure. If this is what you want to achieve, you need to leave all the bad things behind and enjoy your spouse. Make every day count. Make all the good things that happen in your relationship the reason to keep going, while you make the bad ones an experience, and a story of separation. Make every day feel like the day you found out you were in love with that person.

Chapter 1 The Psychology of Sex

The vision and attitude towards life vary greatly according to the person. Similarly, they tend to be different between women and men, which are especially reflected in sexual intercourse.

For her to show a positive disposition towards sex, no matter how uninhibited it may be, she needs to feel desired and excited. If she does not feel desired and stimulated by man, her instincts will be withdrawn. Indeed, due to the disparity of cultural values between them, the woman tends to believe that if it is not required. It must be because she is not attractive enough or she is not a good lover. All this inevitably influences your erotic behavior.

When influenced by society as competitive as the current one and one which gives so much importance to the aesthetic model, her libido usually decreases. This happens because the woman wants to be perfect and if she does not respond exactly to the pattern placed by society, her self-esteem decreases. It is important to be clear that, on the one hand, men also feel insecurity in intimacy and, on the other, that the attraction she awakens does not depend exclusively on the perfection of her body. Sensuality is a sum of factors in which certain inexplicable chemistry plays a primary role.

While a man may seem very attractive to her, it is not always something physical because emotionally mature women tend to lean toward the whole personality. Ironically, men rarely understand this. Contrary to what they may suppose, the woman does not go in search of the most expert lover but of the one who, in making love, makes her feel truly desirable.

Similarly, her feminine sensibility warns her when he goes to the easy stimuli with the fixed idea of penetration without attending to her desires. This causes her to become inhibited, and ultimately, stop participating. To really enjoy sensuality, it is not possible to set aside certain specific psychological aspects since after a difficult day at home or at work, if you are tired and full of tensions, it is rare to have a good disposition for sex. The same happens if a season of stress or emotional conflict is happening.

Climate of Intimacy

To be open to frank dialogue, imagination and fantasy are the ideal elements to create a perfect climate for intimacy between lovers. When two people get carried away by the enjoyment of the senses, natural complicity is born between them which is conducive to erotic play. The woman craves to be perfect and if she does not respond exactly to the established guidelines, she feels low self-esteem. Frank dialogue and openness to imagination and fantasy are the ideal elements to create a climate conducive to intimacy.

Female sexuality has a slow awakening, needs to be stimulated for a longer time, so she is pleased to be in the arms of the sensitive man, who respects her rhythm until passion arises. If the bodies are allowed to respond freely to their desires, to embrace and stimulate themselves without the urgency of orgasm being interposed, they enjoy each and every one of the seasons of pleasure. This climate of intimacy grows surrounded by external stimuli such as a pleasant temperature, a scented atmosphere of incense, or illuminated with scented candles.

All this helps lovers to relax and positively predispose to enjoy each other. Each of the senses is important in the moment of passion: the color of the garments of the underwear or the sheets and other decorative elements excite the sensory world. Like any ceremony, sex requires a stage and rites that enrich it. It requires more and more exciting ingredients to stop it from falling into monotony. Gradually, an intimate culture is born among lovers who, as mutual knowledge grows, feel freer and more eroticized in each new encounter.

In addition to the skin that awakens with caresses, kisses, and rubs that are in themselves, messages of desire, the voice constitutes a vehicle of great sensuality because he and she enjoy creating their own unique language that increases their passion to unknown limits. Women and men do not express themselves sensually in the same way. That is why shared intimacy is the best ally for them to know and acquire confidence in their erotic games, pampering their senses, and above all, telling them what they want to give and receive to feel the maximum sexual pleasure.

Some sexologists argue that the inner frontal wall of the vagina is an erogenous zone, called the G-spot, and it is very sensitive to stimulation and is highly capable of climaxing. However, the idea is not entirely clear, and many women never discover it. Also, the idea that the hymen is preserved whole in virgin women is nothing more than one of many popular myths.

The Female Sexual Map

The genital apparatus of women is mostly hidden, except for the vulva, which is also not visible, since it is inside the thighs between the pubis or mount of Venus and the perineum. Pubic hair, in turn, hides the major and minor lips, the clitoris, the urinary orifice, and the entrance to the vagina. Its location further lowers the knowledge that women have of themselves.

To get acquainted with the genitals, it will be enough to look at them with the help of a mirror and see how the vulva is, what texture and thickness the outer and inner lips have, and what size and shape the clitoris and the cap that covers it is. It will also be helpful to discover the color, touch, and temperature of that intimate area. Some women are excited to see it, which is completely natural and pleasant but, above all, knowing each other thoroughly is the first step towards a healthy and rewarding sexuality.

The Female as Identity

In addition to being a powerful erotic claim, the hair that covers the mount of Venus and the labia of the vulva has the function of protecting the delicate anatomy of the female genitals. The skin of these fleshy lips is similar to that of the entire body. They measure about 7 or 8 centimeters in length. The labia minora are elongated - sometimes very small, sometimes so large that they appear between the exteriors - and their tissue is much more delicate and of a faint pink color. They are very sensitive to manual arousal, hence their importance in sexuality. These labia minora converge on the clitoris.

The lubricating flows that secrete the glands of the female genital area are responsible for their characteristic smell, which often results in great eroticism for men. On the other hand, many women are insecure because they fear it is unpleasant. At its entrance, the vagina is covered by a thin membrane, the hymen, which partially or completely closes it. The idea that this one is conserved whole in the virgin women is not more than one of the so many popular myths. Actually, the hymen, which is very elastic, remains in some sexually active women while in others who have never even practiced intercourse, it can be accidentally broken given its fragility.

The inside of the vagina is shaped like a canal and can be between 9 and 12 centimeters long. Its walls rub against each other, except when dilated during sexual intercourse. It is a humid, warm, and extraordinarily flexible area to allow penetration or the time of birth since during that, it reaches almost 12 centimeters in diameter. Being hidden, it tends to hormones that give the individual aspects of the color of pubic hair to the feminity of the genital tract. Through the fallopian tubes, these are formed from the lips and the clitoris, the depth, and diameter of the canal connect with the uterus, where the fertilized embryos lodge and develop. The uterus can be felt if the fingers are inserted to the bottom of the vagina. A man's penis can also touch it if it is of sufficient length or if the vaginal canal is short.

The Clitoris

A short ligament joins the pelvic bone with a fleshy bump, which is usually compared to a small penis, called a clitoris, leaving it almost hidden between the labia minora of the vulva. The portion that remains insight is the glans, which is of flexible consistency and is pink in color. Due to its vulnerability, it is protected by a membrane or cap that fulfills functions similar to those of the foreskin. Like the phallus, the clitoris has a spongy and erectile tissue inside that fills with blood during arousal. That is why it increases in size when stimulated and presses the vagina during intercourse, favoring that during the penetration, the vagina sensitivity increases. In each woman, the clitoris has a different shape and size. For a long time, it was considered that the length of this organ was about 3 centimeters, but it has been discovered that it reaches up to 10 in some cases. Its function is to give sexual pleasure to the woman and that this, unlike the man, can be multi-orgasmic.

The clitoris is an inexhaustible source of sexual pleasure for women and it is practically impossible for it to reach high levels of arousal or reach orgasm if this erogenous point is neglected. It is she who, in a natural and uninhibited way, must communicate to the lover in what way she enjoys the most since due to her delicacy, too much friction or mechanical movements at this point instead of exciting can end up numbing the area. It is also important to lubricate - with saliva or with the vaginal juice itself - before starting the friction so that the wave of joy increases.

If the woman knows how to guide the lover by teaching him how to enjoy more, by manual or oral stimulation in the clitoris, the frequency and speed with which she wishes to receive it and in what posture it is possible to excite her during penetration, the enjoyment of both will be fuller.

Chapter 2 Sex and Spirituality

The problem with picking and choosing from an ancient text like the Kama Sutra, which is thought to have been compiled in the 2nd century (although it was likely composed somewhere between 400 and 300 BCE), is that for it to mean something you have to take it within the context of the time. In reality, only 20% of the actual Kama Sutra outlined explicit sexual positions and the majority of these that we will focus on were for heteronormative couples (although there are some queer-friendly passages in the text as well as suggestions). The Kama Sutra is compiled as a number of prove and poetic verses and is thought to be attributed to the sage Vatsyayana and most of the text takes into account Indian philosophy and how to live a virtuous life by elaborating on the nature of desire and its effect on our worldly persons.

For our purposes, it's important to analyze our own approach to relationships and love. How do we define love personally? As something physical or intellectual, or both? This, really, is the purpose of the Kama Sutra: to make us think critically and emotionally about our interactions with those we hold dear. In essence, we are trying to achieve a union, and the most direct metaphorical connection to this is the act of sex.

As a physical sort of communion, it is no surprise that it can either bend or break a relationship, and even the Kama Sutra acknowledges that this is something to be aware of. According to their ancient traditions, people were and are guided by energies that inhabit the body – this is not a unique cosmological approach since many societies enculturate the idea of being 'in harmony' with powers or forces that defy the imagination. In the Indian tradition, however, this link between the spiritual and physical is best exemplified by the embodiment of the genitals. In Sanskrit, these were called 'lingam' (for the male reproductive system) and 'yoni' (for the female reproductive system) and were thought to represent the genitals of Shiva and his wife.

Understanding – and not being ashamed – of our genitals, and an appreciation for their uniqueness and for their ability to elicit pleasure in others is a profound and tangible form of happiness. And regarding them (not necessarily as the metaphorical organs of gods, per se) as something sacred is the first step in being able to share the experience of sex with a partner.

How to Get Started:

Before we get too hot and heavy, we want to start slow – sex is not supposed to be a hasty or cathartic act, but something to savor. To this end, foreplay becomes a huge element of the sexual act, helping us to not only become comfortable with our own bodies and the bodies of our lovers but also stimulating physical arousal and fostering a sense of safety and intimacy.

Safety and Security are probably two of the most crucial elements between lovers – if you don't feel safe, if you are stressed or embarrassed, or more importantly if you're afraid of something, then sex can be a stifling and damaging process, and the union we spoke of will not be possible. Let's look at some of the concrete and specific ways we can include foreplay and create a safe space.

> *1. The Kama Sutra Embrace – this should always be the first thing lovers practice,*

and involves touching each other; however the word embrace doesn't just mean giving hugs, it means using your entire body to hold another person. Take turns among each other pressing and touching the other on their body, running your fingers along their arms, across their belly, over their chest, and down their legs. The idea here is to physically map one another's bodies. This helps bring a full tactile awareness to the one being touched but is also a good way to help build trust between partners. You can also try kissing one another, or brushing your lips across certain parts of the body – but the key here is gentleness; let your caresses be as soft as flower petals, and let your lover want more than what you're giving.

2. Kissing – the Kama Sutra is quite explicit about how kissing should be, and again gentleness is the key. The slower you are able to kiss, the longer you can draw out the process of foreplay, and the more

stimulated both lovers will become. This will also heighten arousal and make the actual act of sex all the more pleasurable. This is also, in a way, a sort of test of patience for both parties, and you are encouraged to seek out parts of the body that aren't normally considered "sexy" – for example, try kissing the inside of the elbow, the top of the scapula, the knee, etc.

3. *Using Nails/Biting – varying the sort of tactile stimulus you deliver to your partner is also emphasized. For example, drawing your nails across their stomach, or allowing yourself to nibble parts of the body. Because the mouth is considered one of the most erogenous parts of the body, it is pleasurable for both people.*
Positive Sexual Environments

As mentioned, the Kama Sutra has a lot of chapters designed to elucidate the fact that love is not just a physical act, but also an intellectual and emotional one. While we would like to focus on the physical aspects, being able to develop an environment that is conducive to sexual trust is indispensable. Some suggestions include being able to fill your room with things that both of you love or that you can engage in both before and after – for example, books that you both like, a drawing pad, musical instruments, chess, or other activities that can accompany lovemaking.

It is also important that you both feel comfortable. Creating a 'nest' for yourselves that includes soft blankets, pillows, and fragrant candles can help produce a romantic atmosphere and put you both at ease (especially if you're trying something together for the first time).

Music can also be an aphrodisiac of sorts. But don't worry if you don't play and instrument yourself – having a soft slow-paced instrumental music playing in the background as you engage in foreplay is another great way to ease both lovers into the moment and help keep you at a gradual pace. Remember again, we're trying to savor the experience of one another, not rush through it!

Aquatic Is A No-No?

Another amusing aspect of the Kama Sutra is that Vatsyayana advocated that the best way to learn the following techniques and sexual positions was to practice them in water. There are some obvious logical reasons for this, especially ones that involve a lot of flexibility or strength (such as holding your lover up while making love, all at the mercy of gravity), and quite frankly we think it's a good idea. That said, Vatsyayana went on to clarify that there was a certain unethical or 'dirtiness' associated with copulating in water that tied in heavily to the spiritual and religious tenor of the day – while some of these taboos and customs may not make much sense today, and you are by no

Chapter 3 Prepare Mind and Body for Sex

Creating the right environment and mood for an intimate massage is as important as the massage itself. Being disturbed halfway through the massage or finding out that you are feeling cold or uncomfortable can spoil the experience.

An abandoned or interrupted intimate massage can have long-term effects on you and put you off from trying it again because you are afraid of being disappointed again. It is therefore important that you take the following preparatory steps to ensure you and your lover enjoy a complete, blissful and fulfilling massage session.

Peace and privacy

Make sure that you will be undisturbed during the massage. This means planning and preparing to eliminate any potential interruptions. The last thing you want is to receive a phone call during the massage. So turn off your phone or put it in silent mode. Make sure the place or room is quiet, peaceful and pleasant, and that it also affords privacy. Lock the door and put a 'Do Not Disturb' sign if you are in a hotel room. If you are at home, then choose a time that is appropriate when it will be less likely to expect friends or family to come visiting.

The stereotypical ambiance will mean closing the windows and drawing the blinds or curtain closed, dimming the lights and playing some soft music. However, there are no hard and fast rules to do so. You can leave the windows open or the curtains open, if you want to and think that you will still have privacy. You may also prefer silence instead of playing any music.

The lights are also optional. You may dim them or keep them as usual. Some people prefer to light candles or some incense. Talk it over with your lover and choose what you both prefer and feel comfortable with.

Set the temperature on the air conditioner before you begin. Remember that as the body relaxes, the receiver may tend to feel cold, so don't turn the thermostat too low or the fan too high. At the same time, if it is summer and you are in a place that has tropical weather, then be prepared to sweat. Keep some towels and a jug of cool lemonade or water with some glasses nearby and handy.

Feather the nest

More than music or lighting candles, the most important part of preparing for an intimate massage is to choose the place where the receiver will be comfortable. If you are willing to invest in a professional massage table, that's well and good but you don't necessarily have to.

You can lay a mat on the floor and place some clean sheets or a blanket for your lover to lie down. Though some people don't mind using the bed, it's not ideal nor comfortable for various reasons. For instance, you will be using oil during the massage which may stain the mattress. Another very valid reason is that the surface of the bed is not as firm as the floor and this is important for the receiver's comfort.

Clear a place on the floor and arrange everything required; a mat or a thin mattress, some sheets, some blankets, cushions or pillows, towels, oil and anything else you may need.

It's up to you to lubricate or not

Using oil as a lubricant during the massage is optional. Some people may prefer not to use any oil. Not using oil for a full body massage is permissible but it is recommended that you use some kind of lubricant to perform the Yoni massage or the Lingam massage. Since both these massages involve contact with highly sensitive parts such as the vagina, clitoris, penis or testicles, not using oil or lubricant can cause discomfort or even pain.

If you are using oil, then make sure it is suitable for massage. Some of the most commonly preferred massage oils are almond oil, coconut oil or grapeseed oil.

Use oil that is natural and or organic rather than something that is synthetically concocted or blended. It is also a good idea to use oils that you have tried and tested. You don't want any skin irritation, rashes or any form allergic reaction.

Bath or shower

It is recommended that you bathe or shower before a massage to truly enjoy it. It is also healthy and hygienic to do so. A nice slow warm bath before beginning your massage will help relax the muscles and also make the skin feel supple. You may also consider taking a shower together before beginning to set the mood for intimacy.

An intimate massage session has the power to take you to heights of pleasure you've never before experienced. So prepare well to enjoy the pleasure without any limitations or hiccups. In the next two chapters, we look at some of the most intimate ways to pleasure your lover.

These techniques may seem like foreplay because they involve direct contact and massage of your lover's erogenous zones and sexual parts but it is essential to keep in mind that you don't necessarily need to have a goal of sexual intercourse or orgasm.

These intensely pleasurable massage techniques will enable you to experience intense erotic sensations if you are willing to explore them for their own sake and without any prejudice or preconceived expectations. These massages can help you connect not just physically and sexually but emotionally and spiritually as well.

Chapter 4 Keep Your Enemy Closer

Keep your friends close, and your enemies closer. Men rarely talk about premature ejaculation because this is a direct insult to their ego. But as self-help anonymous groups dictate, the first step to solving the problem is admitting you have a problem.

Premature ejaculation is spilling semen way before you or your partner intended. This may happen shortly after penile penetration into the vagina. In some cases, this happens even before penetration is performed. This may cause dissatisfaction to both partners and when no improvement is made, it may certainly be a cause of problems.

Men of all ages are affected by premature ejaculation. Most men, if not all, at one point in their lives, may have gone through this problem. The complaints seem to arise from different situations and there is no definite cause for the condition. It is believed that the cause is multi-factorial.

Some theories say that it is caused by initial overstimulation and lack of control of it. Others say that it may be due to a lack of practice or long periods without intercourse.

Psychological causes may also play a part. This includes experiences of previous trauma and loss of confidence due to frequent experiences of premature ejaculation.

There may also be relational causes, such as less attraction to your partner. A male who also feels inferior to his partner, for whatever reason, may also exhibit these conditions.

Spiritual and social influences may also cause someone of high moral standards to view sex as a sinful activity and cause sexual problems.

The physical aspect of premature ejaculation is the very last to be investigated once all the aforementioned causes have been treated or ruled out. Physical causes of premature ejaculation are rare. Deeper evaluation may reveal problems in the reproductive system or the urinary tract.

With prolonged premature ejaculation, more severe erectile dysfunctions may occur. As with most conditions, early detection is the key. The earlier you set forth to solve the problem, the earlier treatments and solutions can be made.

The important thing you should note is that premature ejaculation is not a life-long condition. It is transient as it is treatable. Through diligence, healthy living, and proper care of your package, you will be able to control the situation.

Treatments and Drugs

Like most things there are certain options for treatment for premature ejaculation. It isn't the end of the world and it doesn't mean that you have any serious medical conditions. Only a very tiny number of people can actually attribute premature ejaculation to a medical complaint but if you are at all uncertain, you should go and see your doctor. Treatment options include topical anesthetics, behavioral techniques, counseling and oral medications. Do keep in mind that the results are not going to be instant, except perhaps in the case of Viagra or other similar medications, and it may take time to find the right treatment for you.

Behavioral Techniques

Therapy may be prescribed and this will involve a number of simple steps for you take, steps like masturbating a couple of hours before you are going to have sex. This can help you to slow down ejaculation during the actual act and help you to last longer. You may also be told that you should avoid actual penetration during sex for a while and concentrate your efforts on other types of sex play. That can help to remove a lot of the pressure from sex as you won't be expected to "perform" as it were.

Pause and Squeeze

This technique is often touted by doctors as a good way of holding things back and it will involve your partner. It works like this:

- You should begin sex as you would normally, making sure your penis is stimulated almost to the point of ejaculation

- At that point, your woman will need to squeeze your penis at the end where the head and shaft join one another. She should hold the squeeze for a few seconds, until you lose the urge to ejaculate

- Once she releases you from the squeeze, wait another 30 seconds then resume your foreplay. You might find that your penis loses some of its rigidity when it is squeezed but don't worry; once you get back down to the pleasure, your erection will return!

- Again, when you get to the point of ejaculation, your partner will squeeze again

This should be repeated as many times as you feel necessary until you get to the stage where you can actually penetrate your partner without immediate ejaculation taking place. After a while of doing this, you will get to grips, if you'll pardon the pun, with knowing how to stop yourself ejaculating straight away and you won't need to continue with this technique

Topical Anesthetic

These are sprays and creams that contain an agent like prilocaine and lidocaine, agents that cause numbing. If your doctor recommends this course of action, you will have to apply the cream or spray a little while before you are going to have sex, so that the sensation is reduced and you can delay your ejaculation. You can purchase these products over the counter but it is best to go to your doctor.

While topical anesthetics can be effective, they do have the potential for side effects. Some users have reported a decrease in sexual pleasure and a loss of sensitivity and, in other cases, the woman has reported feeling the same thing. Also, if you have to apply these creams a short while before you have sex, it means that you are having to plan it and that means the fun is gone, there is no spontaneity anymore.

Oral Medication

There are a few oral medications that can help to slow down an orgasm from happening but many of them are not actually approved by the FDA for the treatment of premature ejaculation. However, that doesn't stop them from being used and include antidepressants, phosphodiesterase-5 inhibitors, and analgesics. These might be prescribed for daily use or to be taken on-demand, and they may also be prescribed as part of a plan that includes other treatments as well.

- *Antidepressants* – Some men have had great success with using these to delay things a little, simply because one of the side effects of most antidepressants is a delay in orgasm. The most common ones prescribed for this purpose are of the serotonin reuptake inhibitor family – Zoloft, Paxil, Prozac or Sarafem. If these are not successful in helping to slow down the time it takes you to ejaculate, you may well be prescribed Anafranil, or clomipramine – a tricyclic antidepressant. Unfortunately, the possible side effects of nausea, a dry mouth, feeling drowsy and a decrease in libido (not what you want) may be enough to put you off taking this one

- *Analgesics* – Perhaps the better known of these is Tramadol, normally prescribed as a painkiller with a side effect of delaying ejaculation. It may only be given to you AFTER the above SSRI medication has been tried and failed Again, the side effect may be unpleasant enough to make you not want to take it.

- *Phosphodiesterase-5 Inhibitors* – These medications are generally used as a way of treating erectile dysfunction but can also help in cases of premature ejaculation and include Viagra, Revatio, Cialis, Adcirca, Staxyn, and Levitra. Side effects may include flushing of the face, headaches, temporary changes to your vision and nasal congestion

Counseling

Also called Talk Therapy, counseling involves you sitting down with a mental health provider and talking about your experiences and your relationships. The idea behind this is that it can help to cut down the amount of anxiety you feel about your performance in bed and to help you cope better with stress. This is normally used in conjunction with drug therapy.

A Personal Story – How I Dealt with Premature Ejaculation

This the story of how one man overcame premature ejaculation; we'll call him Sam for the sake of preserving his identity. Hopefully, his story will help you to see that you too can overcome this troubling situation. It might also go some way towards showing you that, truly, you are not alone. More men than you realize suffer from premature ejaculation; they just don't talk about it, mainly because of the perceived embarrassment and the stress it causes. Without wasting any more time, let's hear what Sam has to say

The loss of my virginity – and my self-respect

Some people say that too much masturbation, rushed masturbation at that, causes premature ejaculation. While this isn't true of everyone, I'm pretty sure that was at least partly to blame for me. When I was a kid, masturbation was very much a taboo subject and, like a lot of guys, I would rush it without giving it any thought.

I can't blame it all on that. I think some of it comes down to when I lost my virginity.

I was a bit of a late starter, not losing my virginity until I reached the age of 19. I met the girl in a nightclub, she was a friend of a friend and, after the nightclub shut we headed back to my place to carry on with the fun we'd been having that night in the club.

Things heated up pretty quickly and, already pretty damn excited from the hours I'd spent dancing close with her, with all the flirting and the foreplay, we never even got close to having sex the first time – I was just too quick. At that point, I didn't know anything about premature ejaculation, had never even heard of it, but I did think that it would have been nicer to have lasted beyond zero seconds!

At the time I didn't realize it but, in that one single moment, my sexual confidence was knocked for six. In the way that many women do, she didn't let on how disappointed she as and, fair play to her, she tried so hard to make me feel that it was OK. Clearly, though, it wasn't.

Sadly, the second time was no better and, at that point, I was embarrassed and horrified, not just for me but for her too. What didn't occur to me was that this was the start of everything, the beginning of all my anxieties over performance.

And, just to add a bit more fuel to the fire, I now realize that my penis is physically sensitive – doomed from the start.

The excuses, the silence

To my shock and amazement, she stayed with me but over the next week or so, I found out how bad the problem really was. If I waited for 24 hours or more between sex sessions, I was done for, I couldn't last longer than a minute at the absolute most. If we had sex over and over again I would get better although I still never really managed to get over the five-minute mark. And that was only if she was prepared to wait for the third or fourth time that was a bit better.

As the months passed, our sexual relations got less and less. Do you know what the most shocking thing is, though? We never once talked about it – ever

To this day, the most embarrassing thing for me is that I never spoke to any partner about this problem over the next few years and I never did anything about it, either. Not even when I finally took the plunge and got married. Perhaps even worse is that none of my partners nor my wife ever mentioned it either. Well, my wife (now my ex-wife) would sometimes call me a "bastard", jokingly when I came too early.

To be fair, we would talk occasionally about the fact that I would come quickly on most occasions but we never talked about it in a way that would register it as a problem that needed to be fixed. All that happened is, like my first girlfriend, the sex got less and less to the point where it was a rare occurrence.

Selfishly, I turned the situation around and said that it happened because we didn't have sex very often and when we did, I just couldn't handle it. Whilst this is, in a small way, true, it doesn't change the fact that I should have sorted this problem sooner, that it was my problem, not hers.

Ironically, after I split up with my ex-wife (not because of the problems with sex), I could finally admit that I had a problem, a serious one that needed dealing with. The day I admitted it is a day I remember more clearly than the day I finally lost my virginity. It was an awful day as well as being a fantastic day. It was awful because, by admitting that I actually had this problem also made me realize that is should have admitted it sooner, many years sooner. I sat there and I thought about all the women I had left frustrated, screaming silently that I couldn't make it last. How many of them told their friends, people that I used to socialize with?

On the good side, the fact that I had finally acknowledged that I had a problem meant I could take steps to solve it.

Taking the first steps

As a man who spent so many years denying that I had a problem, ignoring it, when I finally did admit that is suffered from premature ejaculation, I suddenly found that I was extremely dedicated to solving the problem.

Obviously, the worst and hardest bit was actually admitting that there was a problem. The rest, all the research and the steps in dealing with it, would be easy in comparison, or at least, I hoped they would. The first thing I did was searched the internet and read up on the subject in men's health publications but, sadly, I found most of the information was somewhat vague. Then I discovered a book called The Ejaculation Trainer.

That book was responsible for two things – it gave me hope ad it gave me homework to do. Apparently, the key to unlocking the problem of premature ejaculation is in practicing lots of different techniques while masturbating and/or having sex.

I discovered that there was no instant cure, that these techniques would pay off but not straight away. There were some tips that I could try straight away though and I did.

The next time I was lucky enough to have sex, I tried to use a number of the instant techniques and, yes, there were definitely a few improvements. It was hit and miss, though – sometimes I found I was lasting quite a bit longer while other times it was only a fraction longer.

The time I tried desensitization products

I never even knew these things existed until I read somewhere that you don't need to use them. Well, of course, that got my mind whirring. I already knew that I had a sensitive penis so it was worth a try, wasn't it?

The first one I tried was condoms impregnated with benzocaine – trust me guys, don't bother. Annoying isn't the word here. I tried a product called Priligy, but aside from the fact that it didn't really agree with me, it just didn't work.

I went on to try out a whole load of creams and sprays but, one after the other, they caused me problems or they just didn't work. The more I tried, the more frustrated I became because nothing seemed to work. Then I found a product called Promescent and, by God, it worked. Only as a temporary measure but it was a good one and, to my mind, a miracle.

So now I had this product that was helping me to last for between 10 and 20 minutes at a time, pretty good for the guy who never got past a couple of minutes before. Time to focus on the natural techniques I had learned to see if I could rid myself of this embarrassing and frustrating problem.

Natural techniques

For a couple of months, I stayed away from the women and kept to myself I needed time to get these techniques sorted and put them to the test. I practiced every single day and also learned to understand both my body and how to control my levels of arousal.

It must have been another two months before I was in a position to have sex again and I could put it all to the test. It was very difficult not to feel anxiety but it was important that I didn't. I had already done quite a bit of research about performance anxiety and I was fully prepared in having to deal with it; it seemed that all of the efforts I put in had paid off.

That first time again can't really be counted as a reliable marker because I'm ashamed to say, I was a little drunk, although this wasn't altogether a bad thing – alcohol does help me in that department! The next day when I had sex again was a different matter – I found that I could last much longer than I ever had before.

But, do you know what the most ironic thing about all of this is? I had come to realize that, by talking about it, the anxiety would be reduced and I would be able to last a lot longer. Believe me, the most awesome moment was when the woman I was with, the woman I had told about my problem, looked me in the eye and said, "trust me, you don't have a problem".

Could I at long last, say that I had overcome the problem of premature ejaculation?

It's an ongoing thing

What I came to understand is that, if these natural techniques were going to work forever I had to keep on doing them. If I slack off, my performance times drop, more so when I have been without a partner for a while and stayed away from women.

I have to regularly practice Kegel exercises or my strength starts to go, as does my control. I have to make sure that, whether I am with a partner or on my own, I take my time so I don't end going back to the bad habit of rushing.

If I chuck aside everything I learned about controlling my level of arousal, about breathing properly about learning when to stop, and all the other important things I learned, and just go at it, the difference in performance times just sucks. There is little I can do about it except for keeping up the techniques and the learning.

And, what doesn't help, I still have a sensitive penis; the likelihood is, it will probably always be that way and, I feel it is because of that, when I am with a new partner after being alone for a bit, that I still have problems.

In all honesty, that is when it is the most difficult to get all of the techniques I learned to work. So, when you have been without a partner for a while and you have had issues with premature ejaculation, it is important to be realistic in your expectation of how things are going to be with a new partner, at least to start with.

The best advice I can give you

If it has suddenly occurred to you that you are not lasting as long as you should be in bed, the most important thing that must concentrate on is focusing your efforts on dealing with the problems. Don't do what I did, don't ignore it, the fact that you have a problem because it isn't going away. In fact, it will only get worse.

Do your research, find out exactly what works for you and never give up. The hardest part is n admitting that you have the problem in the first place; the rest, while not plain sailing, is considerably easier to deal with. Trial and error will play a big part in the next few months of your life but you will get there.

Now I can tell you something. I spent many years studying Psychology and I worked in mental health. So, how did it take me so many years to accept that I had a problem, that it was my responsibility and that I needed to deal with it? The point is, it doesn't matter who you are, it doesn't matter what you do as a job or what you study; the important thing is that you learn from my mistakes and don't ignore it,

Three years later

That was three years ago and, I am ecstatic to report, things are getting better by the day. A time has passed, I have learned to fully understand my body and levels of arousal; I can now determine when I get to the point of overheating and in danger of rushing things.

I can exert enough control over myself now to the stage where I can proudly say that I no longer suffer from the problem of premature ejaculation. 10 minutes or more are the norm for me now, on many occasions I can go for much longer.

Things take a step backward if I am in a high state of arousal and I don't use a condom but I now have a confidence I never had before; I can take full control of my sex life and I can do everything I need to keep things in check.

I don't use any kind of delay spray or desensitizing cream and over the years have come to realize that using natural techniques is the only way to deal with this.

Best advice? Don't hold back, get started on learning how you can control yourself today and learn how to last much longer in bed.

Many of the natural and other techniques that Sam used to help him are discussed throughout this book.

Chapter 5 Reconnect With Your Partner

Whether you've been dating for a couple of months or a couple of decades, it's absolutely typical and solid for sexual longing to rhythmic movement over the span of a relationship. However, in the event that the respite has been too yearning for you and/or your accomplice, you may need some assistance in sexually reconnecting once more.

Life gets occupied. Calendars act as a burden. Also, like most types of self-care, our sexual experiences... the very thing that can be topping us off superior to anything whatever else... regularly gets returned on the burner. By sexually reconnecting with your spouse you'll feel more content every day, your contentions will either disseminate or de-raise speedier, and you will feel all the more profoundly associated with your better half all through your relationship. A sound sexual coexistence is one of the significant discussions that you have with your spouse on a continuous premised... and on the off chance that you've basically quit imparting, your relationship is going to take a colossal hit.

Join with your own body first

Keeping in mind the end goal to have a sound sex drive, solid relationship to your sexuality, and general nice sentiments about your body, it's genuinely basic that you feel associated with your own body.

It's inexorably normal, today like never before, to feel separated from our physical bodies. As a general public we tend to practice less, invest less energy in nature, invest additional time on computerized gadgets, and devour more erotic entertainment than at some other point ever. What's more, as an aggregate result, we frequently feel extremely in our heads rather than our bodies. Without that previous extension constructed between our brains to our bodies, it's hard to have a solid moxie and considerably harder to completely appreciate the sexual delight we're encountering as we're encountering it.

Keeping in mind the end goal to balance this excessively 'in our mind' method for living you can do a couple of things.

– Invest energy in nature. Go sit in a woodland (or in a recreation center) with your exposed feet on the ground. Feel the breeze on your body. Breathe in the aroma of your surroundings. Completely drop into the occasion.

– Activity. Go for strolls. Run. Do yoga. Go to the rec center. Do whatever medium-high power game feels the best time/fun-loving/trying for you. The oxygenation and cell reclamation enhances your sexual pleasure and stamina, as well as it equalizations your invulnerable framework and gives your sex drive a jolt.

– Scrub down. Get kneads. Do anything that makes you feel the physical outer sensation that re-sharpens you to how your body encounters touch. Talking about which...

– Masturbation. Every single awesome beau does. Masturbation is one of the best ways you can all the while re-sharpen to your body while likewise recollecting/finding/refining precisely what sort of sexual incitement you locate the most pleasurable. Put aside standard time to see what you appreciate the most while jerking off (paying little heed to regardless of whether you peak) and you'll see the advantages make an interpretation of themselves into your sexual coexistence in a way that you never thought conceivable.

Uproot any significant blocks through discussion

There's unquestionably something to be said in regards to "interface to begin with, impart second." And generally I concur with along these lines of considering. Be that as it may, if your sexual coexistence has been in a respite for some time (and "a while" can mean whatever you need it to mean) there are likely a few things that you or your spouse need to say keeping in mind the end goal to feel like you can sexually reconnect once more. Possibly there's been an uncertain contention that should be tended to. Possibly there are certain stressors that one or both of you have been juggling and you need an open discussion about it. Possibly you simply need to check in with one another and have a genuine, profound discussion.

Whatever arrives that should be tended to, it likely should be tended to before the sexual vitality can begin streaming between you once more (to the extent that you both realize that it can). Whether you have the conversation(s) in or out of the room is dependent upon you. Wherever you feel the most agreeable, that is the place it ought to happen.

Possibly you have to make inquiries like.

"How have you been feeling about our sexual coexistence of late?"

"How have you been feeling about us of late?"

"Is there any uncertain stuff that you feel like we have to discuss?"

Sparkle the notorious light into the dim corners of the majority of the implicit things between you… and you may be astounded in respect to how the all the more profound, fair truth that is called into the light, the more the sexual vitality begins to stream once more. It's not unprecedented for unthinkable themes to be discussed and after that one or both spouses feel a moment shift noticeable all around that leads them to destroy one another with sexual enthusiasm. I sincerely trust that if individuals all the more as often as possible used the strength that it takes to have the intense discussions in their connections, the Viagra/Cialis/Levitra/E.D. pills business sector would lose 20% of their income overnight. The speediest path to a stone hard erection or a smooth, wet vagina may simply be a genuine, soul exposing discussion about something genuine.

More truth = more sexual stream = more capacity to sexually connect.

Begin with these association works out

Since the significant points have been verbally tended to and managed in a cherishing, empathetic way, we can get to the more physical association works out.

I have found that, for me by and by and for endless customers, these taking after association activities are super effective for helping us moderate down, drop into the occasion, furthermore, reconnect with our spouse in a way that we aren't inclined to doing all the time (unless you've been tailing me for some time and consistently utilize my tips).

7 breath brow association

I have expounded on this one in the past in my article 6 Association Practices For Couples, and it bears rehashing. It's straightforward. You gradually meet up, brow to temple (or third eye to third eye for you all the more profoundly slanted people), and you experience seven rounds of associated breaths. You breathe in gradually together, and breathe out gradually together at least seven times. You do this without talking, and with your eyes shut. This activity helps you truly match up to your accomplice, and it additionally energizes you both to back off and concentrate on your breath. It's a superb activity to use to pick up a clear, moderate snippet of association regardless of what the setting is. I have a few hitched customers who do this activity with their spouse each morning and consistently, as their non-debatable non-verbal check-in.

Nestle for 10+ minutes

Nestling is fabulous. One of the best things that we can accomplish for our sexual association is re-coordinate more touch into our lives. Also, one of the most ideal ways we can do that most proficiently? Rather than flipping through Instagram, checking our email, or perusing our computerized books before we nap off, why not take a stab at organizing developed nestle sessions?

As people, we all ache for touch... and we particularly cherish it from individuals that we as of now love also, worship. So stop your gadgets, set a clock on the off chance that you need to, and snuggle for some time. The cheerful chemicals that get discharged in your cerebrum will help you rest superior to very nearly whatever else you can do before bed at any rate.

Kiss for 10+ minutes

Keep in mind when you were more youthful and kissing was its own prize, and not only a preparatory step that unavoidably prompt sex (as is basic in long haul connections)? All things considered, prepare to have your mind blown. Kissing is still generally as magnificent.

Kissing is a profoundly cozy act, however we regularly hurry through it too rapidly to recollect that fundamental certainty. Investigate your accomplice's mouth with yours. Grasp their face.

Moderate down and completely appreciate that it is so magnificent to kiss somebody you cherish so profoundly. Kissing is a discussion... and it's one that you would prefer not to race through. Certainly. Some touching/grabbing/pounding may normally happen in your 10+ moment make-out session and that is absolutely fine... yet let the kissing become the dominant focal point for some time. You may be amazed in respect to how it's advantages penetrate all through the greater part of your sexual play.

Amplified one-way foreplay

Presently, I don't even truly trust in the word foreplay in light of the fact that it sets up the thought that there is stuff that you do "before sexual play" and afterward the gathered "well done," otherwise known as penetrative sex. I feel that the word sets up an awful outlook for our sexual experiences. In any case, it's still a typical word so I'll meet society where it's at. Much the same as backing off and getting a charge out of kissing is incredibly fun (and profoundly close), having non-hurried amplified, one-way foreplay is likewise fun and profoundly imply. I would even contend that foreplay, in the customary comprehension of the word, is the closest part about sex.

We back off and set aside an ideal opportunity to center the total of our consideration on making our spouse feel as well as can be expected potentially feel... through the utilization of our hands, mouths, toys, and whatever else that we can consider/they approach us for. This is likewise where the last point in segment #1 becomes possibly the most important factor... if our spouses have ventured up the allegorical bat when it went to their own particular self-pleasuring, ideally they'll be sufficiently brave to request precisely what they have to feel the best. Furthermore, if they aren't open to asking, we can either ask them straightforwardly amid the sexual play, on the other hand essentially go off of their non-verbal signals (pacing of breath, development of their body, groaning, and so on.).

Whatever you end up doing in your sexual play, moderate down, take as much time as is needed, have a good time what's more, your spouse's joy completely, and alternate so that you each get the opportunity to concentrate on both the giving and the getting stages.

Ruining sessions

Ruining sessions are as basic as their name infers. You and your spouse alternate gifting one another with a continuous piece of time (30 minutes, 60 minutes, three hours... it's dependent upon you) where you extend your physical and sexual closeness (as coordinated by the beneficiary). It's essentially an activity where you at the same time work on being narrow-minded, while additionally expressly requesting what you need.

Possibly your spouse needs you to begin off with a back rub... or kissing, or snuggling. Possibly they need you to go down on them in a sure position for some time. Possibly they need to have moderate, erotic sex with you while you listen to their most loved music coming through noisy, bass-y speakers. Whatever you do amid your ruining sessions is up to the beneficiary (clearly inside of whatever limits you are both alright with).

Keep in mind, this activity is a safe place stretch for many people (particularly the first or two times that you do it) on the grounds that we're not used to expressly inquiring about what we need in bed. So be understanding and adoring with yourself. It's an activity. It will bring about development (in you exclusively and in your relationship). So set aside your time with it, and give it a couple tries (each) before you choose how you feel about it. In the event that you stick with it, it could transform into the best thing that ever happened to your relationship.

Organize it to keep the energy going

While transient blasts 'DO' convey worth to our connections/sexual experiences (like the burst of bliss/association that you get from setting off to a weekend workshop or experimenting with a ruining session one time), they are still only devices. The way that we genuinely and profoundly shift the nature of our connections (and lives as a rule) is by building new propensities.

Whatever you have found has worked the best for you (from kissing to snuggling to ruining sessions and past) out of the above rundown, talk it over with your accomplice, and make a responsibility to make these propensities a piece of your normal schedule.

Placed them in your calendar. Make your association time non-negotiable. I would suggest a supreme least of once every week (in the event that its different hours long) as far as possible up to each morning and/or night. Nothing matters more than the association you feel with your close accomplice. Such a large amount of your bliss, wellbeing, and professional fulfillment is attached to how cheerful you feel in your home life. So make it need number one and see what happens.

A few individuals believe that putting association/discussion/sex/your relationship in your timetable is un-hot - yet I feel that there's nothing sexier.

What's sexier than demonstrating your spouse "I think about you so much that I need you to take up different time-spaces in my date-book... on the grounds that you're justified, despite all the trouble. We're justified, despite all the trouble. Our association is my most noteworthy need in life."

Our time and consideration are the most profitable assets that we will ever have. So give them unreservedly to your spouse and your whole life will thrive. Furthermore, there's nothing sexier than deliberateness.

Chapter 6 Breathing and Diaphragmatic Breathing

Who doesn't love a good orgasm? There's nothing quite like it. We all seek them out and when we find them, are lost to world - briefly. That said, the other type of orgasm – cosmic, rolling and long-lasting – implicates all that we are and for extended periods of time. There is only one way to arrive at this state of bliss and that is through the pursuit of sexual continence. While this may not be for everyone, it's certainly worth a look. Most of us, I'm sure, will be content with re-lighting the flame of passion with our beloved partners. Some of us, though, once that's occurred, will want to take that passion to the next level, which is more intensely spiritual than any other we've discussed. This level of union is the purest form of worship that can be engaged in. Two bodies joined in sexual union, which doesn't have orgasm as its goal, are experiencing a rare state of extended and limitless bliss few others can attain to. For that reason, I'm including this section on supportive exercises for those of you interested in exploring sexual continence and giving it a place in your sacred sexual practice.

Breathing

Improper breathing represents a disconnect between our bodies and our minds. That's because breathing is something we don't think about. It's an automatic, physical function that we do even in the deepest levels of sleep. Breathing mindfully connects our bodies with our minds and opens our awareness to physical sensation. During sexual encounters, particularly when we're seeking to delay orgasm in the service of reaching toward the divine, breathing is a way for us to control the effect of sensation on our orgasmic potential.

There are two principle methods of breathing that can be helpful in this respect. The first is breathing through the nose. Slow, calm breathing, inhaling and exhaling exclusively through the nostrils, is capable of producing a calm, meditative state and sharpening our intellectual connection with the senses, as we experience them. Your metabolic rate, when using this type of breathing, will also be slowed down.

Breathing through the mouth is a natural way of breathing and usually occurs when our bodies demand more oxygen, or when we're expressing an emotion like surprise, or even sorrow. You'll note that when people cry, the mouth is usually open, especially when crying descends into sobbing.

Breathing slowly and mindfully, exhaling and inhaling only through the mouth, also helps the body to release accumulated toxins and helps to relieve tension in the nervous system. Slowing the breathing allows for the body and mind to be integrated into purpose. By briefly holding the breath following inhalation, consciousness is expanded to encompass sensation.

These two basic types of breathing should be practiced with an eye to making them seem more natural. In this way, employing them as part of your sacred sexual ritual will be less forced and much more part of what you're living as you enjoy your partner in divine sexual union. Perfecting these before trying the technique I'm about to describe to you is highly recommended.

Breathing deeply is also a way of reducing the influence of stress in your life. As most of us have figured out, stress can put a damper on sex. If we're so exhausted by the endless challenges of everyday living, by the time we've come home to our beloved, how are we to even think about engaging in satisfying, transcendent sex? Getting the stress in our lives under control should be part of our breathing practice and one of the many benefits intentionally-practiced breathing offers.

During sex, depending on your level of mastery over your breathing, the most important thing you can do is to be aware of how you're breathing. Shallow or sharp breaths in the heat of the moment may be unavoidable, to a point. But if you're practicing sexual continence, then it's important both partners be fully aware of the quality of their breathing. Monitoring it and ensuring that your breathing is even and slow helps keep your body relaxed. It also ensures that oxygen is being delivered efficiently and filling your blood cells. This keeps you alive to the moment and focused on what you're doing, which assists you to engage the fullness of your sensuality in your ritual sexual practice.

Re-birthing breathing

This technique's intent is to take us back to the first breath we ever drew – the one directly following our arrival on earth. By returning us to that moment, we can experience ourselves on an entirely different level, much more in tune with the cosmos. This method is part of re-connecting with ourselves at the very deepest level.

Lying on your back, with your mouth open, begin to breathe through the mouth, slowly and naturally. Don't force yourself to breathe in any particular way. Just open your mouth and intentionally inhale and exhale through it. Now fill your lungs with air by slowly inhaling. When you're ready to exhale, you'll feel your abdomen deflating naturally.

As you're performing this breathing exercise, think of breathing with your entire body. Intellectually connect those areas of your body you don't normally associate with breathing into the action of your exhalations and inhalations. Visualize your entire body being filled with air, as you slowly inhale and exhale. You will, if you proceed with consistency, take note of a variety of sensations in your body, including tingling. These are due to the influx of oxygen into your system provoked by slow and steady breathing. You will also notice, as you proceed, that your breathing gradually slows even further. You may sense that you are drifting into a somewhat altered state of consciousness (at least, I hope you do).

It's in this altered state, that you'll be able to experience your body and mind from another perspective. You may find that you're able to visualize yourself in the womb, or in another place from the one you're in (astral projection). What you experience with this exercise is the nature of the universe itself, which is a state of tension holding it together. The tension between opposites (as expressed in the co-creative, sacred sex act) is the glue in the universal structure and is also expressed as the simultaneous expansion and contraction of all that is. This is embodied in your breathing. By fully (but naturally) expelling the air from your lungs in this breathing technique, you are both calling on the past (which is present) and pushing it from you, as you breathe. As you pull air into your lungs, you are pulling the change you desire to know in yourself, inside you, distributing it throughout your body. This plays out as a means of becoming the arya you seek to be.

As you breathe, your intellect and your body will work together to identify points at which you've become blocked, or stuck. This will allow you the opportunity to address these threats to your continuing growth. You may also, with practice, arrive at the point at which you perceive absolutely nothing, and have no discernible thoughts and no consciousness. This is the most desired state achievable, using the re-birthing breathing exercise – that of non-being. Only in this state is a true revelation of the self possible, for just beyond it is a place that represents the boundary between our perceptions of life and reality and the truth. That truth is something completely "other"; something that we can't experience in consciousness. In reaching this place, the ecstasy of the truth will open the door to your deepest self-revelation and profound changes that will continue to affect you, long after the breathing exercise has been completed. You will take those changes into the practice of your sacred sexuality and share them with your partner.

In Kama Sutra, sex partners share with one another a divine experience of give and take. This reciprocity should, of course, extend to these breathing exercises. Your partner should also be practicing them.

Chapter 7 Setting the Mood

Creating the right environment and mood for an intimate massage is as important as the massage itself. Being disturbed halfway through the massage or finding out that you are feeling cold or uncomfortable can spoil the experience.

An abandoned or interrupted intimate massage can have long-term effects on you and put you off from trying it again because you are afraid of being disappointed again. It is therefore important that you take the following preparatory steps to ensure you and your lover enjoy a complete, blissful and fulfilling massage session.

Peace and privacy

Make sure that you will be undisturbed during the massage. This means planning and preparing to eliminate any potential interruptions. The last thing you want is to receive a phone call during the massage. So turn off your phone or put it in silent mode. Make sure the place or room is quiet, peaceful and pleasant, and that it also affords privacy. Lock the door and put a 'Do Not Disturb' sign if you are in a hotel room. If you are at home, then choose a time that is appropriate when it will be less likely to expect friends or family to come visiting.

The stereotypical ambiance will mean closing the windows and drawing the blinds or curtain closed, dimming the lights and playing some soft music. However, there are no hard and fast rules to do so. You can leave the windows open or the curtains open, if you want to and think that you will still have privacy. You may also prefer silence instead of playing any music.

The lights are also optional. You may dim them or keep them as usual. Some people prefer to light candles or some incense. Talk it over with your lover and choose what you both prefer and feel comfortable with.

Set the temperature on the air conditioner before you begin. Remember that as the body relaxes, the receiver may tend to feel cold, so don't turn the thermostat too low or the fan too high. At the same time, if it is summer and you are in a place that has tropical weather, then be prepared to sweat. Keep some towels and a jug of cool lemonade or water with some glasses nearby and handy.

Feather the nest

More than music or lighting candles, the most important part of preparing for an intimate massage is to choose the place where the receiver will be comfortable. If you are willing to invest in a professional massage table, that's well and good but you don't necessarily have to.

You can lay a mat on the floor and place some clean sheets or a blanket for your lover to lie down. Though some people don't mind using the bed, it's not ideal nor comfortable for various reasons. For instance, you will be using oil during the massage which may stain the mattress. Another very valid reason is that the surface of the bed is not as firm as the floor and this is important for the receiver's comfort.

Clear a place on the floor and arrange everything required; a mat or a thin mattress, some sheets, some blankets, cushions or pillows, towels, oil and anything else you may need.

It's up to you to lubricate or not

Using oil as a lubricant during the massage is optional. Some people may prefer not to use any oil. Not using oil for a full body massage is permissible but it is recommended that you use some kind of lubricant to perform the Yoni massage or the Lingam massage. Since both these massages involve contact with highly sensitive parts such as the vagina, clitoris, penis or testicles, not using oil or lubricant can cause discomfort or even pain.

If you are using oil, then make sure it is suitable for massage. Some of the most commonly preferred massage oils are almond oil, coconut oil or grape seed oil.

Use oil that is natural and or organic rather than something that is synthetically concocted or blended. It is also a good idea to use oils that you have tried and tested. You don't want any skin irritation, rashes or any form allergic reaction.

Bath or shower

It is recommended that you bathe or shower before a massage to truly enjoy it. It is also healthy and hygienic to do so. A nice slow warm bath before beginning your massage will help relax the muscles and also make the skin feel supple. You may also consider taking a shower together before beginning to set the mood for intimacy.

An intimate massage session has the power to take you to heights of pleasure you've never before experienced. So prepare well to enjoy the pleasure without any limitations or hiccups. In the next two chapters, we look at some of the most intimate ways to pleasure your lover.

These techniques may seem like foreplay because they involve direct contact and massage of your lover's erogenous zones and sexual parts but it is essential to keep in mind that you don't necessarily need to have a goal of sexual intercourse or orgasm.

These intensely pleasurable massage techniques will enable you to experience intense erotic sensations if you are willing to explore them for their own sake and without any prejudice or preconceived expectations. These massages can help you connect not just physically and sexually but emotionally and spiritually as well.

Chapter 8 Spin Your Chakras and Breathe To Ecstasy

There are many practices that you will come across in this book. These practices are fun and you may find them fascinating! These practices include different sounds, symbols and sights that will help you on your journey to ecstasy. You will learn a few techniques in this chapter. You will need to practice these techniques in order to perfect them. The most important aspect of tantric sex is what you are doing this very second: breathing. It is very important that you breathe properly in order to ensure that you are able to attain the deepest level of intimacy and the highest level of bliss.

Focus on the source of your breath

Have you identified that there is a place in your body where your breathing starts? Do you think it is from your throat or chest or stomach area? It is not supposed to come from either of those areas. You have to make the effort to ensure that you breathe from deep within your body. To ensure that you breathe properly, you will have to take a deep breath. Take the breath in slowly and trace the place where the breathing stops with your hand. Then exhale. The next time you breathe you will have to ensure that you take your breath from as low as your genitals. This helps in firing up the energy that you need to have during sex.

Egg to Eagle

This is a great technique to use when you are sitting. You will have to bend into the shape of a ball. When you are bending you have to exhale swiftly. Bring your hands close to your body and place them on the back of your head. Do you feel your back stretching? Inhale and move up slowly into your sitting position. Stretch your hands as far back as you can. Ensure that your elbows are behind you. You should now feel your chest stretching. Arch your back and throw your chest out. You will now feel all the air rushing into your chest. Continue this exercise. You will be able to breathe well after a few repetitions.

The Wells

The aim of this exercise is to take air into your lungs. You will have to take a lot of air into your lungs. This can only be done when you think of your lungs as wells. You will be able to increase the virtual capacity of your lungs. Keep your arms to your side. After you have inhaled, hold the air for a few seconds and blow all the air out with immense force. It should sound like a gust of wind. Then suck in the air by making as much noise as possible. You will make such sound while making love to your partner. Through this exercise, you will be able to ensure that the sounds you make during sexual intercourse are intense!

Chapter 9 Sexual Domination and Submission

BDSM stands for Bondage and Discipline, Dominance and Submission, and Sadism and Masochism. It is also commonly referred to as kink. Let's take a moment to look at what each of these elements stands for.

Bondage and Discipline

This element refers to the restraint and behavior modification of the submissive. Restraining the submissive can be done in many ways and can range for simple ways such a being tied or handcuffed to the bedpost to advanced techniques such as Shibari, which is a Japanese rope form of bondage. Ceiling hooks and bondage cages can also be used. The discipline part of this involves correcting the sub missive's actions with punishments that can be physical and psychological techniques like spanking or erotic humiliation.

Dominant and Submissive

A BDSM relationship comprises of two components: dominance and submission. Therefore, one person plays the role of the dominant and the other, the submissive. The dominant is responsible for dominating the submissive while the submissive gives up control in a BDSM relationship to the dominant.

Sadism and Masochism

This element of the BDSM involves the giving and receiving of pain. The masochist is the one inflicting the pain and experiences pleasure from doing do. The sadist receives the pain and gets satisfaction from it. Sadism and masochism and dominance and submission differ because the former is about inflicting pain while the latter is about control. These two elements are often present at the same time in a BDSM relationship, but they are not mutually exclusive.

Finding a Balance of Dominance and Submission

People who incorporate BDSM into the sex life of their relationship introduce a power play where one person identifies as the dominant and the other as the submissive. As it refers to BDSM, when the male takes the dominant role, this is called male dominance or maledom. Because the word dominant has a masculine connotation, we often associate the role of dominant as one for men. However, there are women with powerful personalities that can handle being the dominant in the relationship. A dominant female is usually called a dominatrix, and she takes the dominant role in BDSM activities.

Sometimes a person acts as a switch, which is someone that can move between both roles. Activities that are common in BDSM relationships include:

- Hair pulling
- Fantasy and role-playing
- Aggressive language
- Spanking
- Flogging
- Fetishes

- Voyeurism and exhibitionism

- Biting

- Using a blindfold.

- Incorporating candle wax.

- Incorporating titles like "Sir" and "Madam"

- Group sex

Couples can engage in just one of these activities or a combination, and the level of kink can range from mild to extreme.

When the term BDSM comes up, most people associate it with Fifty Shades of Grey and Rihanna's song about whips and chains. There is much more to this lifestyle choice, however. There is a lot of misinformation around what BDSM is and what it entails. This is mostly due to the betrayal by the media, where it is mostly shown to be some kind of deviant activity that people with a list of psychologies partake in. This is not the case. BDSM is not a good word for physical violence through sexual means. Most of the time, BDSM is associated with general sadism, being mean, and aggressive behavior. If that is what the couple is into, then that is great, but a healthy BDSM relationship does not automatically operate on this premise.

People from all walks of life practice BDSM, and most of them live quite normal lives. That is because they aim of a healthy BDSM relationship is so that both partners are able to please each other and to cater to their individual kinks. The key to living a healthy and happy BDSM lifestyle is to find a balance between domination and submission. A skillful, caring dominant requires having confidence and being sensitive to your partner's needs. You are not just the dominant because you use a strong tone of voice or derogatory language. While the dominant is in a position of control, it is truly the submissive that has the power because the role of the dominant is to cater to the needs of the submissive. The submissive is the one who sets the boundaries and has ultimate control of what happens in the sexual relationship. It may be that the person enjoys sadism under careful infliction of pain. This does not mean uninvited physical abuse, however. A dominant is someone who is very generous because he sees to servicing his or her submissive desires. A good dominant also places a lot of attention on aftercare, which is the time and attention he or she gives to his partner after an intense sexual experience to ensure that the submissive feels cared for and appreciated. Great aftercare activities include cuddling and conversation about what happened and how the submissive feels about it.

BDSM Misconceptions and Stereotypes

There is a lot of information surrounding this kind of sexual lifestyle, and this section is aimed at helping separate fact from fiction. Here are a few stereotypes about kink and information about whether or not they are true.

- *You need fancy equipment to practice a true BDSM lifestyle.* When a lot of people think of BDSM, they think dominatrix in five-inch heels, a flogger, and Andrew's cross behind her, but practicing does not have to be complicated, nor does it require you to buy any special tools. All you need is your imagination and a partner who is just as interested and eager as you to explore BDSM.

- *People who practice BDSM only have rough sex.* Rough sex is something that many women and men fantasize about but only have the courage to explore with a partner that they trust to care for them and to ensure their safety as well as their pleasure. If that is what the couple enjoys doing, then more power to them, but BDSM does not automatically translate into extreme or rough play. Sometimes, BDSM to a couple means that one partner is more in charge of making decisions in the bedroom.

Introducing BDSM into a Relationship

Most people are afraid to bring up their BDSM fantasies to someone else. Again, this is likely because of the stigma and taboo connotation that society and families have placed around the subject of domination and submission. However, only a strong, well-founded relationship will survive introducing BDSM elements into it. If you and your partner have built a strong foundation based on trust and consideration, you should be able to openly communicate about your fantasies and the possibility of exploring and reenacting them with that person. Make a list of the things that you would like to experience and talk to your partner about them. Find a neutral location to do this so that your partner does not feel pressured to give you a particular response after your disclosure. If your partner is not very familiar with BDSM, introduce the topic in a way that incites curiosity and promotes positivity toward the subject.

To introduce BDSM into a relationship, start small and work your way up to more extreme elements. Small steps can include watching a BDSM movie together, simple role-playing, or introducing a light spank here and there during love making. Try one activity at a time rather than trying to indulge in everything at once. Always remember to respect each other's boundaries and to keep an open field for negotiations. After you two have indulged in an element of BDSM, remember to check in with each other to ensure that you are both still on the same page and to find out what your partner thinks about the experience.

The important thing to remember is that nobody should feel pressured or coerced into doing anything they do not want to do. Both of you should be open to the ideas and approach them with an adventurous spirit rather than a defensive one.

BDSM for Beginners

Getting kinky with your partner has a lot of benefits, but you two can only enjoy these benefits if you begin with a conversation. Both of you need to be educated about what you are doing and the consequences. Communication is vital in establishing dominant and submissive roles and the limits that each person has in participating in this type of sex. Everything that will happen needs to be consented to prior. You do not want to harm your partner or trigger any psychological consequences. BDSM can be a deeply moving and emotional experience for some people, and mental and emotional health needs to be catered to in addition to physical health. The core components of a successful, long-standing kinky relationship are communication, understanding, trust, and patience. Practicing BDSM is different for every couple. Therefore, stop trying to find a stereotypical example to follow. Go with what feels right to you and your partner. Test the waters and keep what feels right and discard what feels wrong.

With that being said, here are a few general rules that you can use to keep your kink safe as well as pleasurable.

Use a Safe Word

A safeword is a word that a submissive uses to let the dominant know if he should stop, proceed, or slow down the action that he is taking. Some elements of BDSM may involve resistance and restraint. This is the only case where "no" might not really mean "no." Therefore, a safe word allows the dominant to know exactly what his or her submissive is feeling at that moment and how he or she should proceed.

Set Hard Limits

Hard limits are activities that submissive or dominant are dead set against doing. Once your partner has disclosed this hard limit to you, you should never, ever venture into that territory as this spells a lack of concern, care, and consideration. By doing this, you can introduce distrust into your relationship.

Ensure That All Pain Inflicted Is Pleasurable

Some people find pleasure in pain, and this is why spanking and slapping are such popular BDSM activities. However, this should be approached carefully so that the pain remains pleasurable and so that it does not introduce long-term or serious damage to tissue or nerves. There is an art to inflicting the right type of pain in a BDSM relationship, and both parties should be educated and informed before indulging.

Practice Aftercare

Sometimes, some people, especially women, experience a condition known as postcoital dysphoria after sex even of the non-kinky variety. This condition includes symptoms like anxiety, irritability, and motiveless crying. This is a common display in submissive as well, and the dominant should cater to this and provide aftercare in the form of emotional intimacy and communication.

How to Tell If You Are a Dominant, Submissive, or Switch

Determining your role in a BDSM relationship is important as it affects the structure of the relationship and how both parties act and react to BDSM stimuli. The dominant is also sometimes called the top and the submissive, the bottom.

Some people think that this is easy to determine based on a person's personality; however, it is not so cut-and-dry. Some people who are outwardly shy and submissive outside the bedroom find the most pleasure in being the dominant in a sexual relationship, while the opposite may be true for people with flamboyant and dominant personalities outside the bedroom. Some people find out they prefer to be submissive in a sexual relationship simply because they are used to wielding so much control outside of that relationship. They would like to turn the reins over to someone else in the safety of that personal relationship and enjoy being controlled. There is a huge sense of relief that comes with knowing what they are responsible for and what other people are responsible for. This person would like to be taken care of and would like to stop worrying at the moment.

The opposite can also be true. Some people who feel that they do not wield enough control in their everyday life such as their work-life find solace in being dominant in sexual relationships. They would like the satisfaction of having someone else's needs and wants placed in their care and to extend on that satisfaction by catering to those needs and wants in the right way.

There is a more special formula for finding out if you are a dominant, submissive, or switch in a relationship. Some people know instinctively which role they will fulfill, but for others, it is not so easy, and the only way that can be determined is by experimentation and experience. Some people try both roles and realize that they are a lot more comfortable in one, while some people realize that they could switch easily between two based on the session or with the partner. Whatever role that you find most comfort in, know that there is no right or wrong. Do not try to put yourself in a box or label yourself as something you think you should be. The beauty of BDSM is that it gives both you and your partner the chance to explore different dimensions in life because BDSM can extend outside of the bedroom and into other elements of a couple's life. It allows both parties to explore their fantasies in a safe and trusting environment. This can only strengthen the connection between the two parties and, as a result, their relationship.

To help make it easier for you to find out which of these categories you may fall into, here are a few personality traits that each of these persons usually exhibits.

Chapter 10 Reel Life to Real Life

Sex sells. That's a fact that some (or many) may not be comfortable with. You can see it everywhere – magazines, TV, advertisements, and movies. While this move contributes to the corruption of minors, it also benefits those in a relationship since it may stir the fire between them.

Majority of films have love scenes where two people engage in coitus. With the proliferation of nudity in media (think Game of Thrones, Californication, and Lady Gaga), couples have been making more excuses to get turned on and make love. Sex scenes in movies and TV also give them another reason (and inspiration) to up the ante in the bedroom.

Stairway to Heaven

Probably two of the most revised movie scenes that involved a staircase were that of A History of Violence and The Thomas Crown Affair. While the sex seemed so good, one may balk a little after realizing how difficult it is to make love on such an uneven and hard surface. But it is possible—and great.

First of all, this sexual position is not limited to the stairs in your home or in the office building (if you're feeling adventurous). This can also be done in the pool if it has stairs built (which is quite common, anyway). Of course, make sure you have the pool all to yourselves or else you risk someone making a sex video of your escapade—or worse, your grandmother walking in on you.

To do the deed, the woman should be sitting on the stair that is aligned to the man's pelvis whose feet are on the floor and his body leaning towards the girl. This is probably on the second or third step. While sitting, the woman moves her arms back and places them on the stair right behind them. This is important for support. She then spreads her legs as the guy leans over to enter her. The man will need his hands for support but if he's strong enough, he can use one free hand to explore the girl's body adding to the sensation. Make the thrusts deep and wild to help her reach orgasm. If you're in a pool, the thrusting motion creates small waves that may help stimulate the girl.

Backstairs Boogaloo

The Backstairs Boogaloo is another sex position that involves a staircase. The girl positions herself fronting the stairs. Her knees are firmly planted on one step while her hands placed on another to keep her balance. The man then kneels on another step below the girl. He then proceeds to take her from behind. Having both knees on the hard stairs may be uncomfortable so some kind of padding may be necessary. Although with the carnal delight brought about by this position and the risk of getting caught (if you're doing the deed in a public staircase), there might be no time to worry about such things. The man may find it easier to thrust with one leg extended down or one knee bent up. For the woman, leaning her chest closer to the stairs may also make things more comfortable.

The Tabletop Position

One of the sexiest scenes in the Richard Gere and Julia Roberts starred Pretty Woman was their characters' sexual tryst on top of a grand piano. The sexual position in question here does not necessarily need a grand piano (though it does add some much-needed elegance and kinkiness). Any high enough surface may suffice as long as both pelvises can be aligned. It's better if the surface is as high as the waist. The dining table, kitchen counter, washing machine, and the boss' office desk are just a few of the things that come to mind.

The Tabletop Position, also known as the Torrid Tabletop, starts off with the woman sitting with her buttocks at the edge of the high surface. In the said movie's case, Vivian Ward was on top of a grand piano in the dark hotel lounge. The guy then grabs both legs in each arm to spread them. She can also open her legs wide by herself to keep the level of seduction on a high. He then positions himself between her legs. Still standing, he then penetrates the woman's vagina and starts thrusting. The lady can lean back and place her hands on the surface. Leaning her head back can also add to her excitement as she cannot see what is happening. She can only focus on the delectable feeling of having sex. The same can be said when she lies down on her back. As for her legs, she can either let them hang loose or wrap them around the guy. The latter is a good way to have more physical contact.

Speaking of physical contact, she can also lean her body forward to be closer to her man. Embracing him or wrapping her arms around his neck is also a good variation of the Tabletop because of the intimacy it promotes. With her legs locked behind her man and her arms on his neck, he can easily carry her from the table and bring her to the bedroom, all while he's still inside her. They can also move on to the Leg Lock position which basically involves him carrying the girl and thrusting into her without the benefit of a table or any sturdy surface.

Another variation of the Tabletop is the Lying Down Scissors. This is basically the same as the Tabletop. The only difference is her legs are extended up parallel to the guy and crisscrossed with one leg over the other. In other words, the left leg is sitting on his right shoulder while her right leg is on his left shoulder. This position creates more clitoral stimulation because of the tighter feel. This is an enjoyable position for both parties.

The Sneak-A-Peek is another position that is derived or started from the Tabletop Position. This time the woman's butt is hanging from the edge and her forearms flat on the surface behind her for support. The guy holds her feet and places them on his shoulders. This position requires upper body strength as the guy has to carry and support the woman. The best part of the Sneak-A-Peak is the guy can actually see everything from where he is – her face, her breasts, her body, and especially her vagina.

This sexual position is a great way to improve any couple's sex life. The simple fact of using other places other than the bed for sex is a surefire way to make things a tad more exciting than usual. The Tabletop Position can be done anywhere in the house as long as the surface is waist-high. For those who want to go to the extreme, the Tabletop is also the perfect position to do in the office, school or any other public place. As long as both parties are good to go and the place is safe enough that you won't get caught (especially if you don't want to spend the rest of the day convincing your boss not to fire you or your local librarian not to terminate your library card), then this position is something you should always have in your repertoire. Where there's a table, there's always a way to have fun and rather dangerous sex.

Chapter 11 Personal Lubricants

Here's where you're going to spend a few bucks, my friends and yes, it's worth every penny. The return on investment for these goodies is about as high a yield you'll get for any investment you'll ever make. And remember what you're investing in – your relationship and re-discovering the passion you've had with your partner in the past. Your love is worth it and your sex life, with the help of a little slippery fun, will be that much more joyous and thrilling.

We've talked about the usefulness of additional lubrication. I know a lot of people will think it's not necessary, or that there are household items which can just as easily be used, but that's not necessarily the case. Don't forget that you have to wash those sheets, towels, the rug, the curtains, the silk boxers and anything else lube comes into contact with. But part of the fun of lubrication is the fact that you have to go out, select and buy it and that such selection and purchase amounts to a pre-meditation of your mutual pleasure. What could possibly be sexier than going shopping together to find just the right lube? A shopping expedition a deux, followed by a private product demonstration. What fun! Let's talk about some of the various types of lube and what they're best suited to.

Slippin' and a slidin' – the lubrication basics

There are so many activities that lube can make better. Any kind of sex act is rendered much more sexual by the simple act of doing it with lube. So what if you don't need it? More is more! This is sex, people and you want it to be as sensual and lascivious, as slippery and as slidey as you can possibly make it. Being conservative about sex is a bit of a contradiction in terms, if you ask me. Go for the gusto!

Like a machine, when various body parts rub together, friction may occur which inhibits the optimum operation of the machinery involved. To keep everything ticking along seamlessly and without operational breakdown, machines often need to be properly oiled. Human beings have similar needs.

While the human body creates its own versions of sexual lubrication (in the uncircumcised penis and in the vagina, when aroused), sometimes, we want a little more of it. Or perhaps, we'd like some lubrication where it's not naturally produced. There are different kinds of lube and this is the first and most aspect of personal lubricants we're going to discuss, sub-genres not excepted.

Water-based

Most people prefer lubricants that are water-based for good reason – they're easier to clean up after. Getting water-based lube on your sheets isn't a catastrophe. Just throw that mess in the wash and be done with it! Same for your body – this type of lubricant washes off easily.

Water-based lubricants are also kind to the skin, as the water used in them is purified. Some lubes, also, can represent the danger of a condom breaking by degrading the latex these are made of. Most of you reading this are in long-term relationships, so I'm assuming you're not using these, but one never knows. It's good information to have at your disposal.

Silicon-based

This type of lube is beloved by many for its texture, which has a sensual, silken quality. Also, extremely good for those with sensitive skin are that silicon-based products that are hypoallergenic. Lubricants made with silicon are also known for their long duration. That means you'll have "re-load" less frequently than you might with a water-based lube.

All that said, the one thing about this type of lube is that it's not advisable for use with sex toys that are made of silicon, as this can cause the material to deteriorate. But take heart, because silicone-based lubricants are ideal for use when you and your love are going aquatic. In the shower, tub, lake, river or hotel swimming pool, silicone-based lubricants are ideal for water sports.

Hybrids

Just like the cars! Hybrids are a little bit water and little bit silicon, which means they can use them in water, too. While maintaining the naturalism of water-based products, they maintain the quality of longer duration that silicon-based products are known for. As with the 100% silicon type of lube, though, these are not good for use with any toys you might have, if you want to keep them in the best possible shape.

Oil-based

Some people really enjoy the sensation of an oil-based lube. Also good for sensitive skin, the heavier quality of an oil-based product can be uniquely sensual. That said, these lubes are not great for use with condoms. Latex doesn't much like oil. As said above, my long-term relationship readers may or may not care about this detail, but it's important safety information I feel it's responsible to include here.

Another important point about oil-based products is that they make a mess. So, if you're a fan, you may want to lay a couple of towels down on the bed before you get rolling.

If you've never used a sexual lubricant before, experiment with quantities. Start with a little and add more, if the two of you feel you need it. A little dab will do you isn't just for hair gel or pomade. This maxim applies equally to lube. It's not exactly cheap, so start small and work your way up from there.

Personally, I'm a huge fan of hybrid lubes for their versatility. My partner and I are water sport enthusiasts, especially when we visit our favorite vacation rental (in an unnamed land), which features a private dipping pool. There's nothing like cooling off after a hot day at the beach with a hot evening in the dipping pool, a refreshing beverage and a side of long duration lubricant. For our toys, though (which we'll talk about shortly), we always use the time-honored water-based lubricant, as we like our toys and want them to enjoy long, happy lives.

My love and I are also fans of any product that warms upon application, as these can add an entirely new dimension to sex play. These are offered over a wide variety of product lines and price points. I suggest you do your research and find the one that's most appealing. Another "best practice" for happy couples everywhere, is carrying portable lubes. These are sachets that can be carried in your wallet or purse and put to work wherever you may be when the mood strikes you. Well worth the small investment required, these babies come in mighty handy in a pinch.

Lube is a chemical substance subject to deterioration in extreme temperature conditions, so like perfume, make sure to store it in a place which is subject to few fluctuations in temperature. You may find that you've soon accumulated a "lube cellar", so give your personal lubricant the respect it deserves and it'll be ready for playtime when you and your love need it.

Where to buy it

You can buy personal lubricants pretty well anywhere, including on the internet. A trip to your local megastore or drugstore could send you home with what you need, too. A trip to Costco could send you home with enough of it for the entire neighborhood! But where's the fun and adventure in such mundane solutions?

I have a better idea!

You and your love will go on a shopping expedition. Every town on the map, these days, features at least one sex shop within shooting distance. If yours is a particularly pokey little town, with only one horse and no such retail outlets, then perhaps a weekend getaway to the nearest outpost of Western Civilization is in order?

Re-discovering the passion you once shared as a couple is all about adventure and this could be one more. Plan your excursion, whether it's in your town, or to a nearby city. Make a shopping list together. Plan your adventure as you would any other excursion.

Once you've decided on the type of lube you'd like to experiment with, write it at the top of the list. I'm about to add to that list, with my personal recommendations of some of the best sex toys and "peripherals". These recommendations are all based on personal preference and incorporate the input of my love, because we've been on more than one such shopping expedition. We love doing this, from time to time, whether in search of something new, to find a specific product, or just to replenish our "lube cellar".

Let's jump into the world of sex toys with both feet. I was once a newbie in the land of the battery-operated sex prop, so if you're shy, I understand. It was, in fact, my adventurous partner who first dragged me into this exciting world and so, I'm returning the favor and inviting you along. Load in those batteries, kids! You're going to need them.

Chapter 12 So you want to be a Superhero?

What do women really want? Well, the answer to that question really isn't all that complicated. Women know when they've pleased a man. They can visually see the pleasure, feel the pleasure and even taste the pleasure they are giving to a man. For men, it's harder to truly identify whether or not the woman they are with has received a great deal of pleasure or any at all, unless of course, she squirts. Women have been known to fake an orgasm just to act like their man has pleased them to that level. But why make a woman fake something when you can actually make her reach that point? Pleasing a woman really isn't that difficult, you just have to give your woman the time and attention that she needs in order to really be able to identify what she likes. DON'T RUSH ANYTHING; MAKE SURE YOU GIVE YOUR WOMAN AS MUCH TIME AS SHE NEEDS!

Many women may be shy or even insecure about what they like. They may have a difficult time telling a man what they want him to do to her. The reality is that while yes, women need to open up and start being honest about this, men also need to encourage the process. Having the initial conversation is crucial. When a woman knows that her man really cares about how she feels and wants her to feel pleasure, she will be more inclined to tell him what will help her feel this way. As a man, you need to tell your woman that you want her to have an orgasm and that you want to pleasure her. This may seem obvious but you must verbalize this wish. Ask her what she likes, do it through text messages or over the phone if it's too difficult in person. Text messages and phone calls have actually helped sexual relationships as they relieve some of the tension when trying to have a face to face conversation about what each individual wants sexually. Actually, text messages can really spice things up and get your girl in the mood. Even a random text message of what you want to do to her can help turn her on. You should not rely to heavily on technology to aid you in your sex life though. At the end of the day face-to-face interaction is the best way to communicate, obviously.

If you really want to make a girl have an orgasm, you have to be ready to try different things in order to help her get there. It can be difficult for some women to have an orgasm, but this is a time when you have to be all about pleasuring her and not yourself. This is difficult for some men. Some men are overwhelmed with the need to have an orgasm and they forget to worry about whether or not their woman received pleasure as well. A real man, or a superhero for that matter will want the woman to have an orgasm over himself. He will make sure that she is pleasured before he allows himself to have an orgasm. While some things are out of the control of the man, such as having a premature orgasm, he will still focus on pleasing his woman first. I've personally had one man ejaculate while he was performing cunnilingus on me. The sound of me moaning during my orgasm was enough to set him over the edge. This just goes to show that sexual pleasure has a lot to do with the mind.

One thing that really encourages most women to have an orgasm is cunnilingus. Women dream, fantasize and think about this often. Cunnilingus for a woman is a time where the woman can literally just lay back and feel pleasure without having to do anything. That being said, this can be a difficult task for a man. The man must try different things with this to really see what his woman likes. Ask for feedback while performing this action, ask her if it feels good, move around, move her legs, pull her to the edge of the bed, try different things until you find the perfect spot. Cunnilingus doesn't have to just be done alone, try using your hands with this as well. When you involve both your fingers and your tongue, your woman is more likely to achieve a full, mind-blowing orgasm. Try one finger first and two if you feel the need, while still maintaining the movement you are doing with your tongue. Really focus on where your fingers are and where your tongue is. While you want to first start by licking all around, you then want to focus on her special spot if you really want her to have an orgasm. Licking that area enough, fast and slow will help her get there. Many women enjoy the sensation of being licked on their anus. Talk about this with your woman and give it a try if you're both think it would be enjoyable.

Once she has an orgasm, you don't need to stop there. In fact, you may even be able to please her twice. Let her cool off for a minute. Right after a woman has an orgasm, she may be a bit sensitive, ticklish even. Give her a few minutes. Try washing your face after this to give her a chance to get cool off and get ready for round two. Washing your face after this will most likely allow for kissing to take place after this is done. This may not be necessary for some women, but others will definitely appreciate it, especially if she's a squirter!

Once you've given her some time, come back and start kissing her. Let her know by telling her that you want to make her have another orgasm. Now, it may be easier for her to have an orgasm by riding you or it may be easier for her to have an orgasm if you're on top. Whatever she wants, give it to her. Before you go in again however, start with more foreplay to get her bodily fluids flowing once more. Start by kissing her softly, kiss her neck, her breasts, even her stomach but don't touch her yet. Let her know that you want her again but give her some time to build the anticipation up again. Foreplay is really important during the time right after she has an orgasm, as it will encourage the likelihood of her having a second orgasm.

Get her in the mood. Gently caress her legs up and down without touching her and let her feel you. This is a soft, sensitive moment, don't rush it. When she feels you, this alone will turn her own. Show her how hard you are. She may even suck you a little but don't let her allow you to orgasm, remember you want her to go again! When a woman goes down on a man this is often a huge turn on for her! Keep in mind, this may be different for all women but many women are incredibly turned on by their man's erect penis in their mouth. When a man is erect and a woman feels this, it will most likely turn her on and she will start to think about what it will feel like inside of her. If you're lucky, she'll kiss you and lick you just enough to get you even harder than you were before. If she starts going too fast and you feel like you won't last long, pull her off of you a little and bring her up to your mouth so you can kiss her. When you stop her from making you have an orgasm, you'll make her want you even more because she'll know that you're really in it to let her feel more pleasure, not just for her to make you have an orgasm and that be the end of it.

Once you feel like she's ready for you, place her in the position that you know will help her achieve an orgasm. This may vary but find the most likely position and go at it. If you don't know, ask her. Straight out ask her where she wants you and how she wants it. She may hop on all fours and show you what she wants. Once again, you won't know unless you ask, so ask away!

Chapter 13 Develop Sexual Intuition

An INSTINCT is a kind of inner force that drives us to act in a certain way to satisfy it ... therefore, the sexual instinct is an inner force, something like an accumulation of energy, which impels us to release it through a practice sexual. While in the rest of the animal species this works exactly like this, in people it varies a little, because the instinct is mixed with other things that influence it.

Thus, among animals, instinct is present as a guarantee of procreation and, consequently, of the conservation of the species, and does not seem to have any other known purpose. Its activation is biological, mediated mainly by the increase of a series of specific hormones, and when it occurs, with cyclical character, gives rise to the so-called period of estrus, which results in the non-deliberate search for sexual partners and copulation, which occurs repeatedly until the activation ceases (the heat).

Among people, the activation of the sexual instinct also has a biological component, mediated by the presence of specific hormones but, above all, by some other factors, such as an image, a thought, an odor, or a slight touch, a dream ... and this is so, because among people the purpose of sexuality is not only procreation but also that of obtaining pleasure, which is produced through the liberation of the energy of which we spoke earlier.

When a man sees a beautiful woman pass by, the reason is hidden. The sexual instinct in man is more developed than in any other animal, so do not say that we act like animals, these normally act in times of reproduction, while a man at all times, because it is more constant since it has much more energy without losing its intensity. In this way it can reach certain sexual abnormalities since its fixations increase, degenerating in its actualization towards any cultural end. Each person is different instinctively, which can be caused by the way of life or how educated. Speaking of sex education, for most societies, in which we live above all we have sought a certain measure of sexual satisfaction, which is one of the social injustices, where a cultural standard required of all individuals for an equal sexual behavior, on which they are based, is good for a person who holds power with a physical constitution that is puny. It is a laugh since the best constituted can suffer a psychic sacrifice. Although it is very difficult that this type of injustice is mostly fulfilled and any moral precept goes down the drain.

It can not be argued that there are people with a sexual instinct that is too intense, that surpasses many, that extreme perversity is manifested and that if it continues in that role, it must bear the consequences of its cultural divergence, otherwise it can reach an inhibition by the demands social results in an unsatisfied satisfaction, by those substitution phenomena caused by inhibition of their instincts, which can cause a series of mental disorders, a continuous internal impoverishment, which will lead to a harmful form for the person.

In the sexual instinct, its purpose is pleasure manifested from childhood, through its erogenous zones and can dispense with another erotic object in the form of autoerotism, so many people with that energy suffer through the culture that repression of the elements of sexual arousal. The sexual abstinence in both sexes has been forgotten, it can be affirmed and argued that there is no harm whatsoever of any person who makes sex before marriage has any consequence, rather what must be accepted is that there is no means to to be able to dominate this powerful impulse that is the sexual instinct, is very strong and less in that fiery stage as it is the youth. To remove that toy takes them as I said before, to a mental disorder, some erase of neurosis, like those suffered by women, but this has changed. In them, this has stopped being "endure" many calamities of man and the roles are reversed in some points, there is no or very little that nervousness caused by marital infidelity, now the nervous man. This severity towards the woman in this cultural exigency is the sexual instinct begins to disappear her desires and fantasies emerge, they do not remain in the neurosis.

The sex trade is broader, more open; Innocence begins to end, temptations are too many. And the impulses got bigger. Abstinence is only left as a word, before it was preferred to virgin women at marriage because the man in his machismo wanted, according to him, to teach them in the trade of their pleasure or to be the first in his life. Some people presume their abstention, but it is a lie, this is supplemented by other means such as masturbation or analogous practice.

This type of activity seems harmless but in the long term can cause a mental disturbance, although beforehand in our culture masturbation is still subject to attack by that existing morality that leads to a custom to keep on that easy path of not fighting for some sexual object where you can develop your energy. That comfort of a small effort that satisfies your fantasies, can deteriorate in your sexual effort because when you want to translate that fantasy to reality it can be difficult.

Men who have this sexual practice, onanistic or perverse can cause their libido to change and at the time of their sexual potential development can be diminished. Just as women who have retained their virginity until marriage, for that sex education imposed by ceasing to have pleasure and when they overcome that artificial delay to their sexual development and reach the peak of their female existence, one can find that relationships with her partner has cooled down a while ago and there is no other way for them to be that unsatisfied desire, infidelity or a kind of neurosis. If these types of people join, what they can cause is a decrease in their erotic faculties, a lack of potential on the part of man and dissatisfaction in both that would weaken the relationship.

An unsatisfied sexual behavior can cause an effect on the children, from an exaggerated tenderness, concentrating on them that need for love which would cause an anticipated sexual maturity. Due to the disagreement of the couple, the child experiences a series of passions such as hatred, jealousy, love which awakens their sexual activity at an early age, which causes a conflict that manifests itself in nervousness that can last all the time. Lifetime.

There is no person who has become ill due to sexual satisfaction, but because of sexual restrictions under the demands of an imposed sexual morality, stagnant libido becomes dangerous and causes illness.

In the same situation, you can not force a couple to a satisfaction through a limited number of populations, as to use that range of ways of making sex that can lead to unfamiliar pleasures, either by fear of another experience or certain complex taxes when you do not want to change, in this aspect you can disappear several things, from the tenderness of the deprivation of sex they turn to another type of illusion, but that usually leads them to that state of domination and deviation of the sexual instinct, promulgating that series of restrictive precepts for society that living in that "double" moral makes believe that they are fulfilled.

Limiting sexual activity increases more factors that disturb the individual's capacity for enjoyment, desire is reduced, fear of life increases and fear of death increases. That sacrifice that is demanded or rather that is imposed by that sexual morality together with other restrictions is restricting freedom and individual happiness.

Chapter 14 Sexual Massages

Massage and sex go together like red wine and chocolate. If you are stressed out and your muscles are tense, blood flow to your genitalia will be compromised, making sexual arousal nearly impossible. To combat this issue, we highly recommend you incorporate some erotic massage into your romance repertoire. A good sexual experience cannot happen unless you wake up your sexual energy and allow it to both flow and build.

However, having a massage manual open on one side of the bed, and stopping intermittently to read a set of instructions is not going to make for the hottest of massages. Anything that takes you out of the moment and keeps you from "Being Here Now" is a turn off to your erotic energy, and stopping to read an instruction manual is definitely an "off."

Unless you are highly experienced at giving erotic massages, even trying to memorize a series of massage techniques is distracting for the massage giver, as you focus mentally on the list of techniques in your head instead of focusing on the touch, taste and scent of your partner. Your partner will feel consciously or unconsciously that you are in your own head, and not totally "Here."

The answer is an auditory guided massage. An audio track that smoothly takes you from one massage technique to another, without the distraction of reading or remembering. A guided massage, so long as it's slow and smooth, allows you to "Be Here Now," and just enjoy and revel in the sensations.

Several years ago we found a wonderful video by acclaimed sexologist Jaiya (yes, like Cher and Madonna, it is apparently just Jaiya), who had created a guided massage video called "Erogenous Zones and Orgasmic Massage" as part of her "Red Hot Touch" video series.

We had intended to describe how guided erotic massage could be used in your love play, and to point you to this great video. However, sadly the video is apparently no longer available (and no, you can't borrow our copy). We then scoured the internet looking for similar guided massages, and unfortunately, everything we found was terrible.

Guided massages have been for us a wonderful way to build erotic energy, and have been part of some of our best sensual experiences. We didn't want you to miss the opportunity to enjoy this, so we decided if you can't find it, make it!

While the sensual but tasteful video portion of Jaiya's video is instructive, we found that it is not really necessary, and that an audio-guided massage is totally adequate. To that end, we made and used our own guided massage audio, and the script to this is found at the end of this book. For us it was even better than Jaiya at building our erotic energy. After all, we made it to our own sexual tastes! You can create your own audio-guided massage, using the script found near the back of this book in "Appendix: Erotic Guided Massage Script" or by adapting it to your own particular pleasures. Simply read the script, slowly and sexily and with the appropriate pauses, into a recording device like your smartphone and then play it back for both of you via a blue tooth speaker and enjoy an erotic massage experience.

The script we have written will result in an approximately 40-45 minute massage, but of course, you can adapt it to be longer or shorter to your pleasure.

Creating your own guided erotic massage will take some effort, but isn't that a great gift to give your lover, letting them know how much you care about their pleasure? You may find, as we did, that just making the guided massage and imagining it as you go is a stimulating experience and a bit of foreplay on its own. We hope you also find that actually doing your own erotic massage leads to some incredible, incendiary sex, just as we did.

One final note on this topic. We know that as we age, our stamina and hand strength can diminish, and for those with arthritis in their hands, this may be especially true. Don't feel like you have to commit to a long full-body session. Even mini five-minute sessions can provide tremendous comfort and pleasure. One area to focus on is the buttocks and upper thighs. We all carry a lot of tension in these areas and helping to ease this will greatly increase blood flow to the genital region, thus allowing for more sexual arousal. One great tip we learned from Jaiya is that the gluteal fold (the crease under your butt cheeks) is actually quite a powerful erogenous zone. Spend some time rubbing and pressing along that area on your partner's body. You may be surprised by the results!

Types of massage to try on your partner

Look into your partner's eyes when you start touching his genitals. Make sure that the connection you made at the beginning of the massage still exists; if it does not, try to restore it by slowing down and asking your partner some questions about what he or she is experiencing. When continuing the genital massage, remember to use your free hand to tease the rest of your partner's body.

Female genital massage

Start by gently rubbing the entire vulva, following with clitoral stimulation, and finishing with internal and clitoral stimulation - do not forget the G-spot!

Vaginal penetration can only take place in case of a fairly extreme level of awakening. If your partner is comfortable, feel free to use a vibrator to help you with the massage.

Male genital massage

Begin by applying a lubricant into the palm of your hands and gently applying it to the penis and testicles. Male genital massage is guided by one essential principle: to slow down and stop or change what you are doing just before ejaculation becomes inevitable. Keep him on the verge of ejaculation as much as possible. Ask your partner to let you know if he is about to ejaculate, which may have the effect of making him enjoy immediately if he is too excited or develops a signal - Change the pace. Play with the brake, caress him, and tickle him.

The massage is nearing completion. By bringing your partner to the extreme limit without allowing him to ejaculate, you prolong the massage and help him to have a more intense orgasm, powerful, if he wishes it.

Sensual or erotic massages

Sensual massage, erotic massage, body-body, and sexual massage are relaxing massages but can go beyond relaxation and well-being. This massage is very different from a traditional massage.

It involves good communication with the other, in a mutual spirit of trust and abandonment. It is sensual in the sense that the gestures are more caresses with a strong erotic tendency. These caresses are worn all over the body, including - but not only - on the genital and intimate parts, for the pleasure and enjoyment of the person who receives them.

This massage is very gradual to appreciate the continuous rise of pleasure better, and intermediate levels are established to slow down and enjoy more of the moment and increase desire.

The pleasure of the person being massaged is the main objective of this massage which can enter the game of caresses not only with the hand, the fingers but also the lips, the tongue, tissues or any other thing contributing to this excitement.

Because some people need to feel the desire of the other to feel theirs better and to express it better, the masseur will let himself be wholly undressed or even suggest to continue with a body-body massage.

Also, some people wishing to go further penetrations will accept the use of their stimulators, their intimate toys or the active participation of the masseur, his fingers, his tongue, his hooded sex, then leading to sex massage.

Body to body massage

This massage is exceptional. It is incredibly erotic and supposes the active participation of the two people who become in turn part of the massage of the other. It is practiced naked, body to body. The body of each is put to contribution, and it is not only hands that massage but the whole body, from head to toe. It implies a willingness to give as much as to receive.

Although the genitals are thus laid bare, it is not a matter of making banal sexual intercourse. On the contrary, the intensity of this massage is stronger when the couples agree to practice it without sexual penetration despite the natural and visible excitement of the moment. This does not prevent the two people involved in this massage to feel desire, or even to enjoy intensely.

In conclusion, on a table nearby, have sweets: fresh fruit, chocolates, and why not champagne in an ice bucket? Choose soft music that invites you to tenderness. If you like the smell, burn incense.

Chapter 15 Mindful Oral Sex

Every man thinks he's a master when it comes to his mouth—whether this refers to his apparent storytelling skills down at the pub or going down on a woman. But in reality, only the men who know that there's no such thing as "being the best at giving head" can lay legitimate claim to that title—because whereas there are basic rules, each woman will get off on a slightly different technique to the next. And even once you've got it right with the woman you're with, sticking with the same old technique time after time is like giving her a red rose every year for Valentine's Day—nice but lacking imagination. I'll give you ideas that can help make the difference between reaching that climax peak and having to remain in the shadows of the mountain, never quite getting to the top.

Finding Your Way

Knowing your route, how long it'll take and what to look for once you've arrived are essential aspects of a well-executed journey—in this section, we'll address ways to make your oral road to her orgasm a smooth one.

Don't go down too early

Heading down there at high speed is like putting her dessert on the table before you've served appetizers and the main course. She may be looking forward to the dessert more than anything else, but she'll want the savory experience, too—it provides a buildup and makes the end of the meal even sweeter. An orgasm is the release of sexual tension, so the more you build that tension, the greater the eventual release will be.

It's also about intimacy; once your head has disappeared down below and she's left with the sight of your forehead for company, it can be a bit disconcerting, especially if you've only been kissing and touching for a short time. But what constitutes a "short" time? That depends on the woman, but here's an easy way to check if she's ready: if you've been kissing her breasts and nipples and she hasn't been pulling you back up to kiss her lips, start a journey with your hands. Let one hand work its way to her vulva—if she's not ready for clitoral stimulation yet, she'll move away or bring your hand back up. If she lets your hand roam free, gradually work your other hand to take over the work your mouth was doing on her breasts, setting your face free to venture south.

Note: As always, sex rules are there to be broken: 95 percent of the time, waiting until she's fully warmed up before heading down is your best bet, but if you're enjoying the kind of red-hot passion session that causes shirt buttons to fly and stockings to be ripped, then rapidly raising her skirt to feast might be just the thing.

When she's not quite to your taste

This is every woman's nightmare, the thought that she might not smell or taste quite right and so you might not be so enthusiastic when you're down there; worse, you might never go down there again.

To avoid any bad feelings, you need to somehow "taste the waters" before it's too late (worst-case scenario is to go delving with your tongue, then rapidly pull away). If you find her smell or taste unpleasant, there's no point in trying to fake it—if she's in any doubt about your enthusiasm to be down there, she'll be wondering what's wrong, which means she won't orgasm. The result? You'll be stuck down there even longer! So use your fingers down there first, then give them a sniff or a lick when you're kissing her neck so she can't see what you're up to. If it doesn't smell fresh enough for your taste, you have two choices: avoid going down there during this bedroom session or suggest a shower. And if you go for the shower option, make sure you make it about getting sexy rather than getting clean: "Shall we do it in the shower?" rather than "Let's go and wash before we get down to it."

What is a normal smell?

It's important here to differentiate between a woman's natural smell and bad vaginal odor. The former is musky, like a more subtle, warmer, and sweeter version of fresh underarm sweat; the latter is like bad breath, rancid and unnatural smelling. The musky odor has a purpose: scientists believe that one of the reasons we still have hair between our legs and under our arms is to capture and enhance our genetic odor—it's a way of giving each other genetic information without having to chat about our ancestry or medical history. Pubic hair also helps protect the genitals from infection by creating a hairy barrier to liquids that could otherwise be absorbed. But don't be duped into believing that removing the hair will remove any odors; far from it, it might make them worse. Removing her pubes could disrupt the natural pH balance of the vagina and can expose her genitals to bacteria that might otherwise be held at bay.

Getting past her hair and lips

Some women are confident enough to spread their legs wide and let you in; others aren't. If you can't get full access or her lips are getting in your way, put your hands to good use.

Getting past her hair and lips

Some women are confident enough to spread their legs wide and let you in; others aren't. If you can't get full access or her lips are getting in your way, put your hands to good use.

Gently slide your hand down her stomach and onto her thigh, easing it away from the other one—this will open up her vaginal lips a little. Now, keep using your hands: place your thumb toward the lower end of her vaginal lips (nearer her anus) where her lips usually sit further apart, and slide your thumb upwards to her belly button, use your other hand to help hold the other lip to one side. This clears the path to her clitoris just like a plow through a field of earth—now follow your thumb with your tongue to find that precious seed at the top of the trough.

Still can't find her clitoris?

If you're licking her all over her lips in an effort to find her pleasure point, don't panic. At this stage she doesn't realize you don't know where it is, she just thinks you're one of the rare (and wonderful) men who spend time exploring and learning about her vulva before heading straight for the clitoris. Some women have huge visible clitorises—the size of a broad bean—others have such tiny ones, you wouldn't bother eating it if it were a pea. But all women have thousands of nerve endings in their vaginal lips as well as that little clitoral button—so explore away, you're getting her well-oiled for the drive of a lifetime.

If you're desperate to get into that driving seat but still can't locate the clitoral gearshift, there is a foolproof way to find it. All women have two outer lips and two inner—they're large and small, fat and thin, never the same and almost never look like the genitals of porn stars who have usually had cosmetic surgery. Start licking at the bottom of her lips, where her vagina is (her vagina isn't the entire genital area, as is often thought, but the "hole" where your penis goes during penetrative sex), and get your tongue between her inner lips. As you slide your tongue from the bottom toward the top—in the direction of her pubic mound or her belly button—you'll reach a point where the lips meet. This is like the corner of your mouth. It's in this area, the "upper corner" of her genital mouth, where you'll find the clitoris.

And if you still can't pinpoint that sexually explosive pea, concentrate your entire tongue on this upper corner—let your tongue flatten against your chin as you grind your face on the entire area. This technique works well for a lot of women because even if the clitoris can't be seen or felt, it's still receiving plenty of stimulation from the pressure your face provides.

When the going gets tough...

Women are, by and large, caring creatures, and so if you've been down there for what feels like forever to you, it's likely she realizes it's taking a while and that'll make her less able to relax...which means she's less likely to come.

Technique

The longest, strongest tongue won't cut the mustard with any woman unless you know how to use it. Rhythm, pressure, speed, variation, and pattern, and all-important saliva, are what you need to be thinking about. And that's what I'll help you do right now.

Easy on the pressure

The clitoris is not a magic button that must be found at all costs and pressed repeatedly until you get her orgasmic bells ringing—the clitoris head is even more sensitive than your penis and some women simply can't handle having it touched directly. It is, however, the key to her orgasm—a woman cannot orgasm without stimulation to her clitoris (scientists believe that even a "vaginal orgasm" occurs through stimulation of the clitoris, but via the "arms" that extend back into her body rather than the head that's visible), but the stimulation needn't be direct. While masturbating, women may use the palm of their hand, a flat vibrator, or even a pillow—this allows for stimulation of the entire area, lips included, without putting too much pressure directly on the clitoris. So how can you simulate that in the bedroom? Easy—use your mouth and chin, and bring your tongue out only for the occasional flat pressure-lick. By using your lips, you can't apply the same zoned pressure on her clitoris as you could with your tongue (try it on your hand and you'll see), but you'll still be providing ample stimulation to the entire region—plenty to bring her to orgasm. Be thankful; pressing your lips into her vulva rather than having to use your tongue on her clitoris will save you a lot of tongue ache. Good news for her, too—that means you'll be able to engage in some post-sex talking.

Practice makes perfect

Keeping up a constant pressure and rhythm is no mean feat—but the tongue, just like any part of the body, can be worked on to become fitter and stronger. Midori, a world-renowned sex teacher, shows her pupils how to perfect oral technique by using fruit as well as a mint candy (you'll have to ask her about that one). She suggests using a plum to strengthen your tongue muscles—you simply keep licking and applying pressure until the skin breaks. Then once you've broken through, you've got to find your way to the plum's stone and get it out! Do that regularly and your muscles will grow to be big and strong.

And, just as you would after eating a plum, lick your lips after going down on a woman, don't wipe. That's the gentlemanly—and very sexy—thing to do.

Forget about licking the alphabet

This old trick has been written about in several sex books and magazines, but I'm yet to meet a woman who says it'll bring her to orgasm. There is a small possibility that she'll climax by having the alphabet licked onto her clitoris, but chances are it will be interesting, exciting even, for no more than a half a minute or so—as a teaser—quite quickly it will feel rather frustrating, like being in bed with a man who has to change sex position after every thrust. Keep the alphabet trick for times you'd like to play with her or get her aroused, but don't rely on it to bring her to orgasm, as you're unlikely to succeed.

Use your hands, too

Ever enjoyed a woman's hands squeezing your behind while giving you oral? Ever reached climax as she's played with your nipples while sucking you? Ever been sent over the edge as she's handled your balls while going down? Well, what a coincidence—women also like to be touched when a man goes down on them. Trouble is, most men (and women when the roles are reversed) are so focused on the task in hand—their tongue and lips and her lips and clitoris—that they forget she even has a body with plenty of other erogenous zones that will bring her to a more explosive orgasm sooner.

Try any of these hands-on approaches:

Start at the bottom. Grab her behind to give yourself better access and extra stimulation power—you can push up as you lick down, maximizing the effects of your tongue or lips.

Find her breasts. If you have long enough arms to play with her love pillows at the same time as giving her oral, you'll be rewarded with plenty of brownie points.

Press on her mons pubis.

That's the bony pubic area above her vagina. Don't do it hard, but if you pull the flesh back here you expose her clitoris and many women really enjoy the sensation.

Don't forget her hands. Grabbing her hands is a nice intimate thing to do when you're giving her oral, plus it also gives you extra control—you can pull her body down onto your face if you have both of her hands in yours.

Techniques to bring her to orgasm quicker

Use one of the following moves when you go down on her, but don't forget to experiment: try variations of each and make up new techniques!

The no-move move

Simply hold your tongue firm and let her do the moving and shaking. As sex therapist Dr. Ian Kerner puts it, "A flat, still tongue is one of the most underestimated oral-sex techniques." And he's so right. If women most enjoyed flicking, darting tongues, they'd invest in a lizard—have you ever even seen a sex toy designed to look like one? No. That's because they prefer a firm, even pressure. Hold your tongue and you'll hold the key to her orgasm.

Chapter 16 Alternative Sexual Experiences

For most people, threesomes, bondage, and anal sex only happen in movies. They don't have to be sequestered into the fantasy realm. With some planning, you can make your anal sex, bondage, or threesome a very sexual reality. Here is how.

Threesomes

If you have a partner that you are comfortable with, you need to pick your third partner carefully. It is a lot more complicated than staying away from best friends or ex-lovers. Relationship and sex experts say that finding one person in your friend group that you aren't that close to but is open to having a threesome. If you choose a stranger, you don't have to worry about long-term attachments, but you do risk not being attracted to the person you are getting ready to have sex with. There are also some safety hazards to take into consideration like sexually transmitted diseases.

If you are single, try dating sites that cater to people that are looking for multiple partners like

POF. This also goes for Craigslist. Craigslist has a tendency to attract some weird people so you might want to FaceTime with them or meet them in person in a group setting first. There are some other sites like 3nder and FetLife that are interesting. You could always go to your local sex toy store and talk with people there. You could ask the people who work there or the owners what happens in the community and you might even find some fliers for other clubs or parties.

It doesn't matter if it is two women and a man or two men a one woman, it is totally up to you either as an individual or couple. Male-female-female is most common since guys are as open-minded about being with another man. With that said, women shouldn't cave just because her partner is forcing his preference on her.

If you haven't discussed this with your partner, you might need to suggest watching a movie about threesomes before outright asking your partner about having one. Once you see their reaction to the movie, you can ask them if they have had one or would be interested in having one.

If it goes well, you might casually ask them if they have anyone in mind to be their third. If you both agree to the person, then you need to approach them in a way, so you don't scare them off. Ask them casually like, "Hey, we think you are cool and fun. We would like to have a threesome, and we think we would have a lot of fun with you. Would you be interested?" If you already know the person, let them know that this will not change the friendship in any way. If it is someone you don't know, take time to get to know them first. Go out to dinner or drinks to see if you have a connection with them and feel like you can trust them.

Don't worry so much about asking. Most people on the receiving end will feel flattered.

You need to set some ground rules well in advance. You could think about taking sleepovers, oral sex, kissing, or possibly penetration off the table. Don't worry about taking activities off the table will make the experience worse, it could actually be more exciting without actually penetrating.

If you are in a relationship, you and your significant other could set up safe words or phrases you could use if things start to get too intense. Let the third person know they can speak up if they ever feel uncomfortable.

There are some things you need to have on hand. You are going to need plenty of condoms. If the man is penetrating each woman, he will need to take the condom off every time he changes partners. If he doesn't, he is exposing them to viruses, infections, and bacteria. Sex toys, lube, and toy cleaning wipes need to be on hand for wetness or added sensations. Toys need to be wiped down between partners, so you don't spread germs.

It is all easier said than done. Don't over-think things. Begin with a glass of wine and some appetizers. Start talking, and this will usually lead to flirting. Somebody will make a move in no time.

Massage is a good way to get intimate. There are massage candles that turn into an oil when blown out. This can be used to give a body rub that will set the mood.

The actual three-way needs to be organic. Maneuver, touch, and move any way you like. If you are a dominate person, take the lead. If not, let yourself be led and do what feels natural.

For some positions, the man could lay down on his back and receive oral sex from one partner while the other woman sits on his face and gets oral sex from him. A different position is one woman lies on her back while the other one lies on top of her. The guy penetrates the top woman doggy style, and the women can play with each other. Another option is to arrange everybody in a circle, and everyone performs oral sex on each other.

There are plenty of places to put mouths, genitals, and hands. If there is a free tongue or hand, find a place to put it.

Threesomes will take longer than normal sex, so you might need to change things up a lot. Guide your partners into ways you would like to do. Pay attention to any changes in the other's body language, sexual cues, and breathing patterns. Use movements to guide them, no words.

If it seems like someone is being left out, reach out and begin to play with them. This will help them to jump back in action.

You will need to figure out what you are going to do after the action beforehand. Let the others know. You might want just to say goodbye then, cuddle up for a while, or just hand out. Just remember to talk about what is expected of everyone, so no one is surprised later on. If a sleepover is planned, the third party needs to know in advance so they can pack an overnight bag.

Bondage

If bondage is new to you and your partner, bring up the subject gently, so they won't freak out. During sex, begin by pinning your partner's hands down and telling them that they are now at your mercy. Let this be a starting point to the conversation about pushing the subject of bondage more.

Blindfolds are a great place to start since they don't feel as strange as handcuffs might. Not being able to see will help some get rid of their inhibitions. Take turns blindfolding the other and then treat them to sensations like, kissing, tickling, lightly scratching, and licking your partner in various places, so they don't have a clue as to what is going to happen next. This will mirror the sensations that happen when tying up your partner.

Before you bring out the handcuffs and ropes, you must choose a safe word if things start getting too intense for the submissive. Try the word yellow if you want the dominant one to ease up but not stop. The word red shows your partner that you want to stop completely. The safe word should never be stop or no since saying these things gives the dominant the right to override your protests. Getting your demands overridden is part of the fun of being out of control.

You should only try bondage with someone you feel 100 percent safe with. Now, set a timer for 30 minutes for your first session because it will be extremely intense. Don't use gags or blindfolds for the first few times. Just try tying up the submissive partner, so you learn to read each other. Do not ever leave a person that is tied up alone.

If you think you are ready to push the envelope, start by using a soft rope or silk scarves to tie up your submissive partner up with in different ways. Allow the dominant to configure the rope into a figure eight that goes between the breasts and behind your back. This will push up your breasts and accentuate them. A different scenario has them stand with their arms at their sides and wrap the rope around the torso, so their arms are tied down. Just be creative, let the rope twist over their body any way that feels right. Touch them sexually with your fingers as you pull the rope across and through their body parts. When you finally have them tied up challenge them to escape. Stay away from the neck area. If you decide to tie their ankles together, be sure they can't fall. Never, ever use bungee cords, these will snap and hurt your partner. Don't tie them up too tight. You should be able to slip a finger between the rope and their body. They shouldn't feel any numbness or pain.

The handcuffs you decide to will help to set the tone. Metal or leather will make you feel like a badass where a fuzzy pair will have you feeling playful. Begin by binding your partner's hands together either in front or behind their backs. Move on to a position where they are secured to the bed with their arms up and out to the sides. Never use cheap costume handcuffs. These can tighten and hurt your partner. Don't use stocking as these can cut into the skin.

The dominant partner needs to move into things by starting out sensual and sweet. Think about kissing softly and slowly. It is extremely hot being tied up but yet being treated very tenderly. As the game progresses, the dominant one can bring out their inner tiger.

For another naughty twist, wrap up certain body parts in plastic wrap, like around your hips and breasts. This plastic drives him wild since he will be able to see but not touch you. When you have him good and worked up, allow him to have his way. Have some blunt-tipped scissors near so they can cut you lose.

Another hot idea is to tie your partner up with toilet paper. Be sure to twist it to make it stronger. Tell them they can't break free and then tantalize them until they can't stand it. When they rip loose, then you can punish them.

If you want to take it up a notch, try using a spreader bar. It will hold your partner's legs apart so you can have your way with them.

Role-playing can help transition into bondage. A few fun games are: pirate/princess, prison guard/prisoner, cop/robber, burglar/defenseless housewife.

The biggest part of what makes bondage so pleasurable is the aspect of not allowing your partner to have pleasure. If they are tied up, begin by slowly stripping in front of them. Let them watch as you touch yourself. When they are begging you to touch them, begin by slowly stroking their most intimate parts and then penetrate them slowly. Tell them that they can't have an orgasm until you tell them to.

If both partners agree to be both dominant and submissive, switch between these roles, and you will be amazed at what will get you going.

Anal

Of all the numerous sex acts, Anal remains the most misunderstood. Anal sex is not the first thing when you think about mutually pleasurable things you want to do with your partner. The urban legend states that "Guys want it since they think it is tighter than a vagina. They have seen it in porn, and women use it as a bargaining chip for special occasions."

Quite frankly, that is pure crap. A lot of women do it just because they like it.

The main thing other women want to know is will it hurt?

All women will agree that yes, it does hurt the first few times. The main thing to remember is to relax. Don't think about it. Prepare for it. It won't be as bad if you begin with lube and fingers. Widening the hole before penetration can help it not hurt as bad.

Why do you want to do it?

Mostly because it is considered to be taboo and naughty. Some do it to impress the guy they are with after a night of partying. Having anal sex when you are extremely turned on is more pleasurable. Some women can have an orgasm during anal sex. The ones who do orgasm during anal, say it is more intense than a normal orgasm.

Who wants it more, the woman or man?

Most women say that their men were the ones who initiated anal sex. Most women concede due to the fact they don't want to hurt their men's feelings. They don't want their man to think they aren't into them. Some have been lucky, and it was mutually wanted. Most men are infatuated with anal sex and butts.

How does it feel the first time?

It is very weird. It is very tight and unpleasant. It is a bad cramp. Just like you are stretching a muscle that has never been used before. If you can make yourself relax and be prepared, it will be better.

What will it feel like after you have done it for a while?

It makes you feel like you are completely full. Very intense. You learn to adjust just like you did with normal sex. With time, you know what you are going to fill and learn to enjoy it. It won't hurt as bad since you aren't as nervous. The initial penetration will always feel weird, but once you get going, it is enjoyable.

Will it ever feel good?

If the person you are with lets you control the force and speed; it can be quite pleasurable. It also depends on the size of the man's penis. If you can combine it with clitoral and vaginal stimulation, it can feel great.

Is waxing a necessity?

No, most decent guys don't care what a female looks like back there. If you feel more comfortable, then, by all means, go for it.

How soon into a relationship should it happen?

If the guy has a fetish for this sort of thing, it is really hard to hide, and he will bring it up right away. Most will wait six months or more until you have thoroughly enjoyed each other in all other intimate ways.

To lube or not to lube?

If you don't want it to hurt and feel horrible, lots of lube is needed. They type is up to you. Use whatever you have on hand or your favorite. If you find yourself out of lube but have coconut oil on hand, that works just as well.

Will you bleed?

You shouldn't bleed as long as the guy takes precautions and uses lube. If he forces himself into you, it is possible.

Do you need to protect the bed with towels?

Anal sex isn't messier than normal sex. If you are a squirter, or just get extremely wet during sex, then use a towel.

What is the cleanup like?

There isn't any cleanup. Just the normal lube and wetness. The condom is the only thing that needs to be taken off.

Are there certain positions or angles to try?

Most say the doggy style is the easiest and most convenient. Some women find it pleasurable with the girl on top so she can control the pace.

Are condoms still required?

Absolutely, condoms are still and will always be a requirement.

Can you have an orgasm from anal sex alone?

Usually not. If you can stimulate the clitoris along with anal sex, you will probably have an orgasm. Don't worry about it if you can't. It is all about what you feel with your partner and how they make you feel. Just enjoy yourself and have fun.

Chapter 17 Would You Ever?

Sex is an endless kaleidoscope of possibilities. Just when you thought it was all getting a little tired, along comes another wrinkle in your sexual world, to shake things up again.

A wrinkle, or a kink?

Ah, there's that word. Kink is not all whips and chains. Kink can involve fetishization of certain types of clothing, or body parts, or even household objects. (Stop looking at the blender like that). Kink can be role-play, or public sexual behavior. It can be lots and lots of different things. For as many people as there are in this world, there are different types of kink and you know what? With willing partners, it's okay.

Sometimes people are awfully shy about admitting to a kink or fetish. That's because we live in a judgmental world. Something I've learned in my life, though, is that those who judge you are the people who are most likely to have a closet full of secrets; things they kept hidden, out of shame. But their shame is not your problem. Only your shame is your problem and the fact is that kinkiness is the human condition. There's nothing to be ashamed of.

Role play

You're a superstar. You know you are. You and your partner are the same people every day, doing more or less the same things. Sometimes, when the moment's right, it's kind of fun to put aside our day-to-day personas and be someone else for a little bit. At least, I think it is. My partner does too.

We were on vacation at an all-inclusive beach resort when we found out just how much fun role-play can be. We spent that vacation mostly recharging our batteries, poolside. Cradling cool drinks in our languidly lazy (and sun-browned) mitts, we were as indolent as the day was long, refusing to budge, except to dunk ourselves in the pool momentarily, or flag the waiter down.

And it was that waiter that broke the camel's back. My partner, much to my chagrin, couldn't keep her eyes off him. I admit that he was a pleasant-looking guy (OK, he was built like a brick outhouse and had dimples you could stick your finger in up to the first knuckle). Finally, after observing her eyes peeping out over the top of her sunglasses to bore holes into the guy's ass as he walked away one too many occasions, I got a little testy.

"I can see you, you know." I snorted, sarcastically. "You're not invisible!"

Naturally, my partner pretended not to know what I was talking about, directing her attention back to her pulp fiction, poolside reading. As for me, I sat there turning the meaning of my partner's ogling ways over in my mind. After doing so for the better part of the afternoon, I began to formulate a plan.

When it was time to return to our room to shower and get ready for dinner, I pretended to have an errand to run. I wandered around the grounds of the resort for about twenty minutes and when I felt enough time had elapsed, returned to the room. Knocking on the door, I called out, "Room service!"

When my partner arrived at the door, she found me there, frosty cocktail, replete with paper umbrella, on a tray I'd managed to convince one of the guys at the swim-up bar to lend me for the occasion. She'd just gotten out of the shower and had come to the door wearing a towel.

"Oh, pardon me ma'am! I'm so sorry to disturb you." My eyes roved up and down the length of her towel-clad body, as I said this, lingering on her breasts.

My partner's eyebrows shot up, as she cottoned on.

"That's no problem. Do come in". She pulled the door open, still hanging on to the towel. Closing the door behind me, she gestured to the table in the sitting area. "You can put that over there". And so I did. But when I turned around, my partner had dropped the towel to the floor at her feet and it was on.

Without so much as saying a word, I had become my partner's dirty little fantasy, come to life in our hotel room. It was as easy as paying attention to what was going on right in front of me and transforming it into an experience we could share and enjoy together. This is where putting aside uselessly hurt feelings comes into play. Why should you be hurt or even mildly annoyed that your partner sees other people as attractive? This is just a human thing and an indication that your partner is, in fact, still living!

Don't get angry. Get creative. Take that attraction and make it a game you can both get off playing. That's how the smart folks do things.

Bondage

A little light bondage can be very erotic. It just depends where you're both at, as to whether this option is going to work for you. I'm not talking about heavy-duty dungeon play. Then again, that might be your thing (which is another book, entirely). I'm talking about light restraints around the wrists and possibly, the ankles. This can work for either partner. Have a little chat. Find out if this is something your partner may like. I've found that springing things on my partner can work either for or against me, so once again, knowing your partner well is your best sexual tutor. You know who your partner is better than anyone. Let that knowledge be your guide.

Your visit to the sex shop can encompass this aspect of sex play, too. There are even kits available, which include everything from feather ticklers, to satin wrist restraints and blindfolds, to kinky little whips made of soft, non-threatening material. Perhaps making a gift to your partner of one such kit can break the ice. If such a presentation concludes with something else getting broken, there's your answer.

Spanking

Spanking is becoming an increasingly popular activity for fun-loving couples. As with everything else in this book, its two-way street and one which both of you can enjoy giving and receiving. You may want to incorporate it into your role play, with one of you playing the principal to the naughty school girl/boy. Lights! Cameras! Action! You may even need costumes.

Spanking, though, needn't even incorporate any elaborate scenarios, or equipment. The flat of someone's hand and a naked bottom are quite enough. When incorporated into your sex play, a little slap on the bum can be powerfully erotic and you may find that you both become rather fond of the activity. The trick, of course, is knowing when you've gone a little too far. It's important, when engaging in any activity involving restraints or BDSM (bondage, domination, sadism, masochism), that you're both invested with the ability to stop the action if it's going beyond what you're willing to indulge. That means employing a safe word.

A safe word is what you say when you don't like the direction the action is taking. It has to be a word that neither of you would normally say in the course of your love play. For example, "Pythagoras" is a rather good one. Also appropriate might be a word like "cumberbund" (it's not as though either of you is going to be wearing one – generally speaking). Having an agreed-upon safe word in place can also be fun at parties, when you're both ready to leave for the evening, or if you find someone to be a terrific bore, but don't dare say as much to his or her face. You can always explain it away as a type of Tourette's, if it comes off as too "weird".

Chapter 18 Conclusion

What a wonder sex can be for a loving couple. When both partners are actively engaged in keeping the flame alive, sex can be the glue that binds them together. When we let that flame die, for whatever reason, our lives together lose something. We become roommates who used to find each other attractive, once upon a time and perhaps forget how that happened.

It can happen to anyone. It doesn't mean there's something wrong with you, or your partner. Letting the fire go out happens to most people, over the course of their relationships, but I'm here to tell you that the condition is not permanent. With some genuine commitment and sustained remedial action, you can light it up again and it won't even take that much effort. It just takes commitment, dedication and the love that's already there, between you and your partner.

That never went anywhere. That love is still there. It's like gasoline, waiting for a match to be dropped on it. Re-learning how to physically express your love is something the two of you can not only talk about, but do. You can do it together. If only one of you is coming along for the ride, then maybe the writing is on the wall. I'm the type of guy, though, who genuinely believes that if the love is real, then the sex is not dead forever. It's just taking a nap and needs a wakeup call.

With your unique, combined creativity as a couple, every day is going to be an adventure. Your willingness to explore and to rediscover the people you fell in love with, will have you falling in love all over again. There was a time when you couldn't keep your hands off each other and that time can be now, if you're willing to do what it takes to make it happen.

My partner and I, like almost every living couple, has been there. We've let the flame go out. But because we know each other so well and because we love each other so deeply, we've been able to not only revive our sexual relationship, we've been able to make it better than it was, even in our earliest days together. As we've grown together we've become stronger and more fully rounded human beings. Experience has taught us many things, as it teaches us all. That's the part about getting older that's beautiful. Life teaches you as you move through it and all that learning can enrich your lives together, emotionally, sexually and spiritually.

Your relationship was born in passion. There's no reason to believe it's not still there. In fact, believing that serves as the cornerstone rediscovering that passion, together. If your love is real, it was built to last and something built to last is worth keeping in the best shape you possibly can.

While life can throw us curveballs, wear us out and squash us down, our response to those challenges is what really makes the whole affair worth living. Being who you are together and who you've always been as a couple, is a shared adventure and sexuality is an important part of that. Whether you're young, old, physically unencumbered, or disabled, your sexuality is an integral part of your humanity. Living that out in all the fullness and joy sex brings to our lives is your birthright and your gift to one another.

I hope you've enjoyed this open, high-spirited discussion about re-discovering sexual passion as a committed couple. More than that, though, I hope you take what I've written here to heart and that you and your partner can put it to the right kind of use – re-igniting the passion in your relationship. By doing that, you can be a light to other couples out there who may be floundering. The quality of your life has changed because of your dedication to each other, you'll stand as an example to others that love is not disposable. It may change, over time. But it's something worth defending and something worth spending the time to reinforce, by giving ourselves fully to each other. We were born for each other. Let's remember that, and live out our love with our bodies, minds and spirits. Let's be the promise we made to one another in the very beginning.

May you re-discover your passion for each other and live as lovers, always.

SEXUAL INTIMACY

A guide to explore desire and sex game for couples, sexual fantasies in marriage and same-sex couples. What women and men really want from sex. Tips, massage, positions

DONNA DARE

Description

Finding time to spice things up in a relationship can be difficult and it takes work. If you want to keep things fun and sexy then you must put in the work. Trying new positions and incorporating new sex toys will keep things hot and heavy between you and your partner. Learning about each other and finding what feels good and what turns each other on is crucial. Taking a trip to a local sex shop or surfing the net for new sex positions is a great way to eliminate the boring sex life that you may have and create a better sexual experience for the two of you. Try new things! This may be intimidating at first but once you become more comfortable with each other it will be much easier.

The fun in having sex involves getting to know each other, your bodies and what feels good for the other person. When you are able to provide your partner with an immense amount of pleasure, this feeling alone is a turn on. Watch the facial expressions of your partner as you lift them up, bend them over, and straddle them or whatever else you do to make them feel good. Allow this moment to turn you on. Most of all, have fun! Sex is a sensual moment for two individuals, but it's also a great way to release stress and feel good. When you have an orgasm, you release tension. Let go of daily stress by making it a point to have sex a few times a week. Make time for this! Great sexual relationships take time and commitment to the task at hand. The task of providing pleasure for another individual is a great thing, but it's also an experience that will open new doors for new ways of receiving pleasure and fulfillment from your partner.

This guide will focus on the following:

- How to communicate with your partner
- Developing your sexual relationship with your partner
- Clearing the decks for sex
- Explore him/her body
- How to give an erotic massage to help increase intimacy
- Unlocking intimate capacity through synergy
- Spicy and dirty talk
- Masturbation
- Orgasms

- Sex toys: what choose for him and for her
- Using props during sex
- Sexual and aphrodisiac food
- The intricacies of pleasure and orgasms
- The most intimate positions for couples... AND MORE!!!

Introduction

A good lover is one who is willing to give her pleasure and who enjoys feeling how desire grows in her. He is attentive to her reactions, without assuming that what has made her or another woman enjoy before is a kind of universal recipe that will always be exciting. In general, it is the one who is sensitive to know how you want to be stimulated, in particular.

Although there are clear responses of desire with direct contact in the erotic points, female psychology can be governed by rejection when the caresses are mechanical, or if they perceive the lover's hurry to erotize them and accelerate the moment of penetration. It leads her to think that he only wishes to stimulate them in search of his own pleasure.

Being more flexible than men, they launch themselves into new games and fantasies, so when they are the ones that are stimulating them, they quickly learn to satisfy them; but they expect and need him to do the same. The ideal lover is the one who is able to notice the subtle changes in the feminine mood. There are women who carefully choose underwear as a claim of seduction and get frustrated if he only notices but doesn't comment. The woman has a more developed feeling of erotic correspondence, so she knows that pleasure does not depend on the sensual capacity of one of the lovers, but on both.

What makes her sexual desires grow more is that as her desire and arousal increase, he should make her feel special and desired. For her, the small details are as important as the big gestures in any sexual encounter. Their morbidness wakes up to situations that escape the routine as when they are caressed while still dressed or half-undressed. Situations that are set aside from the bedroom, moments that remind them of their first sexual scuffles or when lovers run the risk of being surprised. Their fantasies are also triggered if the caresses are not predictable and mechanical friction in the breasts or vulva are avoided. This sensitive mode of the approach causes her to intensely see the stimulation of the erogenous points and begin to crave contact.

One of the attitudes that the woman values and that makes her sexual cravings grow is that, as her desire and excitement increases, he makes her feel that she also enjoys, prolonging the stimulus for her to enjoy. In certain men, impatience is noticeable or they seem to get bored if the woman is slow to get excited, acting as if they were spectators waiting for penetration to begin. This can cause the woman's libido to retract.

However, the most important thing a good lover should know is that the woman is different in her sexuality, more complex and much more subtle. A direct stimulus in the erogenous zones and the enjoyment he obtains through penetration is enough for him since his sexuality is more direct. It is easy for him to reach an allegory. She needs, instead, the mystery and the display of imagination because she does not care about the number of orgasms, or sexual athletics, but the degree of eroticism.

Learning to Touch

Touching the lover for the simple pleasure of doing so, feeling his reaction and perceiving the touch of firmer, elastic or tender skin, awakens perceptions that move, disturb, or excite. But above all, touching is the intense enjoyment of knowing each other without having the precise objective of intercourse or orgasm.

The big secret is to turn the touches into a purpose in themselves. Turn it into a creative game, free and without rules, in which everything goes. There are no allowed or prohibited areas. The flexibility and disinhibition that this seeks are difficult to equate to any other form of knowledge. It is the purest enjoyment that pleases the sensitivity and the exciting territory of the skin.

The Active Role and the Liability

The pleasure of being touched is not less than that which is felt by caressing the lover. Therefore, the ductile and natural exchange of roles brings a playful aspect to eroticism. It is intensely sensual to assume an active attitude seeking to stimulate the other, who gives himself to the pleasure of caress enjoying the situation joyfully. Likewise, the inverse attitude is equally exciting. In this way, not being aware or being routine in the role that is assumed allows each encounter between lovers to contain a subliminal expectation.

She intertwines her arms around his neck or waist, supports her hips while standing and facing each other, playing an active role and conveying her need to feel him very close, as well as being tightly embraced, trapped, and protected. Although the active role is usually identified with masculinity, the truth is that this depends on the psychological profile of each person, whether man or woman.

Self-Carry

The woman, no matter how liberated, finds it difficult to stop associating the caresses in her own body with masturbation. He also has a hard time doing it in front of his lover. Stroking for pure pleasure is the first step to discover new sensations and in every inch of your body.

In the beginning, the caresses should be soft and slow. The arms or legs are a good starting point. The skin will respond to the touches expressing, in its own way, when it needs the rhythm or intensity to vary. Then different types of friction are experienced and alternated: with the open hand, with the fingertips, with greater depth, as if there were small taps, with the knuckles, the back of the hands, with the nails or running with tissues of various textures such as feathers, velvets, and silks.

Awakening the Sensations

Once the game of caresses begins, they become combined, form a chain, and respond to the rhythm that flows freely. He is going to touch the breasts or the back, but he grazes the neck by chance and that changes the planned route. He hears a murmur of pleasure that ignites her and feels the promise of enjoyment offered by that point to his hands, his lips, and his tongue. To her, that exciting contact encourages her to respond by stroking his body or shaking it to feel it closer.

He kisses her softly and affectionately. He only wants to comfort her but she incites him by kissing him, biting, and sucking his mouth. Once the instinct is triggered, it does not resist and descends through the excited body to more vulnerable points that await its touches with deep anxiety.

Imagination is a good ally to transmit caresses to certain unusual body parts, which is sensual contact, offer unknown pleasures. Feel the firmness of a knee stroking the soft inside of the thighs, the nipples sliding down the belly or the female back, the hand that, without stroking, encloses the pubis and the entire vulva in a tight and warm wrap intimate, are some suggestions which will help you to not fall into repetition. The true awakening achieved by touching is one of the plateaus of enjoyment, a point in the path of pleasure.

Be Acierated from Front and Backs

Sometimes, caresses begin with clothes out of which, little by little, one strips off. The nakedness communicates between the skin of one and the other a contact which is not only sensual but also of a great emotionality. Some parts of the female body are largely forgotten, usually because of the positions that are adopted. It is the case of the back that, due to the multiple nerve endings that run through the center and along the spine, when touched, responds vividly. She is lying on her stomach and her back is in view; he caresses her with alternating touches. Worrying about aesthetic perfection often limits the pleasure you feel, given the possibility of feeling rejection from it. Actually, a man does not give much importance to this issue, but his sexuality awakens first and that sets some unsaid parameters. Imagination is a good ally to transmit caresses to certain unusual body parts.

The most exciting sensations wake up when a caress or casual touch finds an exact point of sensitivity that remained hidden and that, once stimulated, provides a surprise and unexpected pleasure. He caresses those with the hands, then rubs it with the knuckles, inserts taps, kisses, and licks between the shoulder blades, in the center, until reaching the edge of the waist, without advancing in principle beyond. She moves sensually, feels relaxed, and stimulated at the same time.

He continues to play downstream, palpate the buttocks, and traces its contour with an unprinted finger to caress with passion. It is as if he is drawing its shape. He then reaches the legs, passes the fingertips lightly through the soft inside of the thighs, and reaches the calves, caresses them, and then takes the sensitive toes one by one and kisses them warmly. If she seems pleased and he notices her relaxed body, he gently incorporates it until she is seated. Then, standing behind her, he caresses her breasts, initiating the soft and very slow touch at first without directly looking for the nipples. Their movements are enveloping and rotating. You can also simply hold the breasts between the palms of the hands.

After a prolonged and intense caressing session of him, she wishes to participate by caressing herself or returning the caresses. If self-stimulation is reduced to a simple sexual discharge alone, sexuality is impoverished.

Chapter 1 How Communicate with Your Partner

It is true. Communication is the key to any successful relationship. Especially when it comes to something like Kamasutra. It is the duty of each partner to ensure that they are satisfying their lover, but it is also their duty to let their lover know how they are feeling.

Humans are not minded readers, and often times do not know what you are thinking. You have to be open with your partner and allow your partner to be open with you. Otherwise, you will have some serious issues. A lot of times people are not open because their partners shut them down, and get angry at criticism, so they feel that they are not able to be open. You have to encourage communication both in and out of the bedroom.

In the bedroom, make your partner feel comfortable with vocalization. If they are nervous, let them know that it is not silly, and you like knowing that what you are doing feels good, or if it doesn't feel good, you want to know so that you can make the proper adjustments. You should also lead by example. A lot of times one partner is very vocal, while the other is silent, you should both be vocal. Do not be afraid of shouting or screaming in pleasure. Also, do not be scared to tell your partner what doesn't feel good. You can make it less harsh by asking them to change something nicely, rather than saying that hurts. This way there is no killing of the mood.

You also need communication in your everyday life as well. When your partner upsets you, you should tell them rather than bottling it up until it becomes a fight. You should also tell them if they are doing something you like. Too many times in the real world, everyone talks about what they don't like, but no one talks about what they do like. Yet in the bedroom, it is the opposite. You should definitely find a balance in both.

Communication is a necessary part of your everyday life. Even if it is just talking about your day. Many relationships fail because there is not enough communication to keep the passion alive. You want to tell your partner everything. When they ask how your day was, it is because they want to know. They do not want a one-word answer such as "good." When they ask you, be free with the information. Tell them every little boring detail, and then ask them about their day. Revel in what they are saying to you, even if the words are unimportant. Your lover will be happy knowing that even if they had a really boring day, you want to know about it. Things like that are the little things that make the world go round, and indeed make a relationship work. Communication is a show of love, and it will help keep your love strong. Use it to its fullest power.

Chapter 2 Developing Your Sexual Relationship with Your Partner

It can be intimidating making that transition from simply flirting into a full-blown sexual relationship with your partner, but it is good to know that for most couples, the more sex that they have the better the relationship becomes when it is based on mutual respect trust and love. Before having sex with anyone, it is important that you are completely comfortable discussing sexual affairs with that person and that you are 100% ready for that step. Do not allow yourself to be pressured into making any decisions because the only right time to move to that stage in your relationship is when both people are on the same page about sexual intimacy.

When Is the Best Time to Have Sex for the First Time?

This is a complicated question, and the right answer varies from person to person and relationship to relationship. To some people, the answer is the very first day that they meet someone. To others, that right answer maybe a few weeks or months into dating someone. Not before marriage is the right answer to other people. While the answer to this is complicated, one thing for sure is that sex should not be engaged in unless both parties are completely ready for the act. This is especially true if you are a virgin and have never had sex before.

Tips for Having Sex with Your Partner for the First Time

The initial stages of exploring your sexual attraction to your partner can be filled with excitement and adventure as you learn what each other's turn-on are, explore each other's bodies, and tap into each other's sexual fantasies. However, before you just dive in, be sure to have a discussion about sexual boundaries, meaning what you both are okay with engaging in the bedroom. Both of you need to be frank and open about what works for you sexually and what does not. By eliminating the worry that your partner might unknowingly go into territory that you are not comfortable with, you can both simply enjoy the moment and being together.

The first time that sexual penetration occurs in a relationship can be particularly anxiety-provoking for some couples. It may be the first time that you completely bare your body and, therefore, your vulnerabilities and insecurities to that person. However, no matter how intimidating that moment may be, it should be something that is supremely enjoyable for both you and your partner. To ensure that this is the case, I have compiled a few tips to ensure that your first time goes as smoothly as possible.

- *Get into a relaxed state of mind before the date.* While the first time can be a spontaneous event, most couples know exactly when the first time will be. Being tense will make this an awkward and probably unfulfilling event. Therefore, prepare yourself mentally with simple meditation or yoga techniques to soothe any nerves that you might have. Think of it as a pre-sex warm-up.

- *Wear clothing and underwear that makes you feel sexy.* Knowing that you look good will feed your self-confidence at the moment. This does not automatically mean that you should wear thong underwear or exaggerated lingerie pieces. Sexual attractiveness and comfort should go hand-in-hand. Make sure that you look good *and* feel good in what you are wearing.

- *Do not focus on your appearance.* Sometimes we focus too much on how we appear during the active sexual intercourse such as wondering if a position flatters us or if the lighting compliments us, and we don't focus enough on how we feel at that moment. Remember that your partner is with you at that moment because he or she is already attracted to you. Just focus on your enjoyment of the moment.

- *Take your time and make-out first*. Anxiety and pure horniness can make you feel like you need to rush to the main event for the first time but resist the temptation and allow the tension to build with a pre-sex make-out session. Since this is your first time with your partner, make it something that you will remember forever. Savor each sensation and every moment. By taking your time and making the moment last for as long as possible, you both get as aroused as possible and are both more likely to orgasm from the session.

- *Bring protection.* Do not just leave it up to your partner to take on the responsibility of ensuring that you have protection. You are both equally responsible, and if that person happens to not have any, you can be assured that you have got things covered.

- *Do not be afraid to voice your needs and ask questions.* If your partner is doing something that you really like, do not be afraid to tell them so. The same goes for if they are doing something that you do not like. Instead of being worried about if your actions are pleasing to them, simply speak up and ask. It is important to build your sexual communication skills right off the bat in any relationship, and it is no different for your first time.

- *Laughter is good.* Sometimes sex can be funny. Maybe it is an awkward position, bumping your foreheads together, or the dreaded queef that arouses a moment of hilarity. Whatever it may be, do not be afraid to laugh. Not only does this beat awkward and not put too much pressure on the moment but it also helps bring you two closer.

- *Do not bring up past lovers or past sexual encounters*. I think this goes without saying but most people do not like being compared to someone's past sexual partners even if the comparison is done to show that they are better. By doing this you will only make the moment weird, so do not do it.

- *Do not focus on your orgasm.* This is especially useful advice for women. This is not to say that orgasming is not important; however, putting too much pressure on reaching it can be the reason why it does not happen. Do not focus on the big finish but rather on enjoying yourself at the moment.

Masturbation for Couples

Another first that many couples encounter in their sexual relationship is shared masturbation. Before we get into how masturbation can improve your relationships, let's tackle a few myths about the act. It is simply not true that masturbation will:

- Cause you to go blind or make your eyesight go bad.
- Cause the male penis to shrink in size.
- Make you go insane.
- Cause cancer.
- Give you an STD.
- Cause you to become homosexual or adopt a homosexual lifestyle.
- Hinder your social and emotional development.
- Make you sterile.
- Make you unfaithful.

I do admit that some of these myths border on ridiculous; however, many people do believe in them, and it is important that we educate as many people on sexual topics. It is true that masturbation can be harmful to a relationship if it is done in the wrong way. You will know that you are doing it wrong if:

- You have to hide the fact that you do engage in masturbation from your partner.

- You look forward to masturbation more than you look forward to being sexually active with your partner.

- You substitute masturbation for intimacy with your partner.

- You masturbate to the point of self-injury.

- Masturbation interferes with your personal and work life.

- You feel shame regarding the act because of religious beliefs, family views, or media messages.

- You have tried to stop masturbating at such a high frequency and have been unsuccessful at stopping or decreasing the amount of time that you spend doing it.

In such cases, while masturbation can indeed affect your relationship, this is an issue that needs to be dealt with individually. It is a great idea to seek the help of a therapist and enlist the help of your partner so that you can get the help you need.

The negative outcomes of masturbation on a relationship can include the promotion of feelings of inadequacy. This is a consequence when one partner hides that they engage in masturbation and the other party finds out. The person who finds out may feel that their partner is bored or unhappy with them as a sexual partner, and this may give rise to insecurities. It can also give rise to distrust. If indeed one party was engaging in masturbation in secret, the other party may feel that they cannot trust this person because they have kept such an important aspect about themselves secret.

As you can see from all of the negative incomes above, masturbation that is done in secret and without communication with the other party is detrimental to a relationship. By being open and honest about your needs and exploring the satisfaction that masturbation can bring, you can open the door for an even healthier, more active sex life with your partner. Again, it all starts with effective communication.

Getting the courage to masturbate in front of your partner can also be intimidating because of body issues and revealing so much of yourself to someone but masturbating together, which is also called mutual masturbation, can allow both of you to bare it all physically, emotionally and mentally at the same time.

Benefits of Mutual Masturbation

- You can sate your need for sexual satisfaction before you are ready to be completely intimate.

- It is a great stress reliever in long-distance relationships.

- It allows you to be sexual even if you cannot engage in penetrative sex for reasons such as risky pregnancy, risk of STD infection, or disability.

- It allows you to spice up your sex life by trying something new with your partner.

How to Masturbate Together

The first thing to do is to get comfortable. Find locations and positions that allow you to have eye contact. A particularly receptive position is to have the woman straddling the man's body. This gives both parties a full-frontal view of what is going on with the other as they masturbate at the same time. In addition to allowing each party to touch themselves, this position is great for simple touches to each other's face and chest. It also allows kissing which can increase the feeling of closeness and deepen the connection at the moment. There is also nothing wrong with giving each other a hand. The man can offer clitoral and G-spot stimulation while the woman strokes his erect penis and testicles.

There is no right way or wrong way to proceed with mutual masturbation. Do whatever feels right and good to you and your partner. If you are looking for a few ways to spice things up, here are a few ideas:

- *Add sex toys to your mutual masturbation fun.* Common sex toys include vibrators and dildos, but sex toys are not only limited to being used on women. Some men find that they like the sensation of vibrators against the skin. There is even a special sex toy for men called a stroker which fits into the hand and goes over the penis and acts as an artificial vagina. When using sex toys, be sure to use plenty of lubrication to avoid uncomfortable friction. Water-based lubricants are normally compatible with all sex toy materials.

- *Talk dirty to each other.* Dirty talk does not have to be complicated. Simply telling your partner what you are doing and how good what that person is doing feels increases the sensuality of the moment. Adding instructions can also add a dynamic of power play that some couples find very stimulating. Adding talk of fantasy is also considered dirty talk.

- *Try phone sex or do it over webcam.* This is a particularly useful tip if you are separated from your lover. Long-distance does not have to keep you from enjoying each other, and mutual masturbation is a great way to keep the sexual tension alive and well between the two of you.

- *Watch porn together and masturbate.* Many people find that watching certain porn videos arouses them, so why not use the on-screen stimulation to masturbate together? Reading erotica out loud to each other is a great alternative to this.

Oral Sex Techniques

Now that we have gotten comfortable discussing masturbation and using our hands to please each other, let's take a look at how we can use our mouths for mutual satisfaction as well. Oral sex is a beautiful expression of desire and love and can be one of the best ways for increasing sexual intimacy with your partner. This section is dedicated to helping you increase your oral sex skills to drive your partner crazy with lust and desire.

There are some general rules that apply no matter who is on the receiving end of oral sex, and they are:

- *Educate yourself.* Before you engage in oral sex, you need to be familiar with the names and functions of common sex organs such as the clitoris and the perineum. Oral sex will be a whole lot easier and more enjoyable for both parties if you eliminate ignorance.

- *Be clean as a common courtesy to your partner.* Ensure that your body and mouth are thoroughly cleaned as well as keeping facial hair and pubic hair trimmed and neat to avoid abrasion.

- *Keep bedside essentials handy.* Oral sex can be a messy affair, so it is a good practice to keep clean up devices such as tissues or wipes handy. Other items such as lubricant, hair ties for keeping long hair out of the way, sex toys, and a glass of water for the inevitable dry mouth or dehydration should be kept close as well.

- *Remember to reciprocate.* Both parties should be able to enjoy receiving oral sex, so remember to reciprocate the pleasure that your partner gives to you and vice versa.

Chapter 3 Clearing the Decks for Sex

Sex isn't something you should just "count on". That's one thing my love and I have learned over the years. For us, the initial fire hasn't so much gone out as it had to be domesticated and kept in its proper place. To be truthful, that's because we entered into our relationship with a strong awareness of how tenuous love can be. We were both committed to maintaining the quality of our bond and that meant a frank and open discussion about our sex life together, once the initial madness of love had subsided.

You know what it's like. You can't keep your hands off each other. You can barely be in the same room together, without "going there". People yell "Get a room!" at you in the street, because you're always smooching (and proudly so). Exhibitionism and day and night eroticism fuel the early bonding of all couples. Keeping that feeling alive, though, when life interrupts your mutual sexual reverie, can be a demanding and serious undertaking.

Tempus fugit (time flies)

It's no secret that the fast-paced nature of life can get in the way of our sex lives. This is especially true if you have children (babies and very young children, especially). The demands of child-rearing present their own challenges. But that's not really the focus of this book. Let's focus on ways and means of making sure you're not putting your sexuality on the back burner out of sheer laziness, cavalier neglect, or just exhaustion.

Sex in a long-term partnership can dwindle in many ways and being aware of that effect is one of the most important steps you and your partner can take to stop it from happening. The first defense against heterosexual bed death is honesty. Being honest with your partner when you sense you're neglecting each other's physical desires is key. Getting offended is a bad sign. It means you're not fully engaged and that your ego is more important to you than the health of your relationship.

Another is not making time, but taking it. Grab time by the face and make it your bitch! It's your time. It doesn't rule you. You rule it. Stop saying you don't have time. You do. You just need to move the furniture around a little to make space for sex. Sure, it's work, but any marriage/partnership requires some of that. Those who don't think that's true are probably best suited to "confirmed singledom". If you're not willing to admit that your relationship has been forged between two fallible humans, you probably should go it alone. Denying that your sex life is waning, being egotistical about approaches from your partner to address it, or laziness about doing the work involved, are not going to help. These attitudes are going to lead to the revolving door.

I'm speaking from experience. That experience, while not the most fun part of my life with my beloved, has been formative and has made me a better partner, overall and certainly, a better sex partner. So how did that experience inform us both? How did we put a stop to protestations of there never being "enough time for sex", or of being "too tired"? Most importantly, how did we do it without blaming each other, or being hurtful? Here's what we did.

Making time your bitch

My love and I are both hardworking people. One important decision we have made in our lives was not to have children. That's not for everyone. I know. But it's a decision neither of us has ever regretted, so that factor has never been a question. But work and its demands, social obligations, family and all the myriad things in life that keep us busy can build up, exhaust people and push sex to the bottom of the list. It happened to us, about four years after we began co-habiting. That's not bad, as it's a generally accepted reality that most couples experience a diminishment in sexual intensity after the first two years together.

That's right. Only two years. So if any of our relationships are to last more than two years, it's highly advisable that you take what I'm going to tell you next seriously.

At about the four-year mark, both my partner and I had continued with our careers, working hard as the General Manager of a large chain store (me) and the proprietor of a marketing consultancy (her). We were doing well, economically. We were prospering. But it was clear that focusing on our respective career paths had taken its toll. We were both tired. But more than just tired, we'd become so comfortable in each other's presence that weren't being as sensitive to one another as we'd been in the earliest layer of our relationship.

"I miss you," she said one day, over a hurried breakfast. We'd started to make a point of rising a little earlier in order to enjoy some time together in the early morning, regardless of how little of it there was.

"Me too," I replied, wistfully. We knew right then that we needed to act. My partner's tentative approach didn't lay blame. It didn't accuse. It was a simple statement of fact that got my attention. After about eight months of slow drift, with the television set numbing us into complacency, she had realized that someone needed to say something. One of us was always falling asleep in front of it – in our holey sweatpants, of course. Whoever remained awake would rouse the other before crawling off to bed – to sleep. We'd been using fatigue as an excuse to avoid the question of physical intimacy. But what was really in the way was the pacifying soporific effect of the TV.

So we turned it off for good. We loaded that sucker into the back of our SUV and drove it to the nearest Sally Ann. It was one of the best things we ever did for ourselves. Maybe some of you don't want to hear this, but that box is sucking the sexuality right out of your relationship. The time you spend staring at that thing is better spent with your partner. Some of that time is sex time. Interested now? I thought you might be.

Neilson, the company that monitors television viewing habits and derives ratings from them, conducted a study in 2014. This study revealed that the average American between the ages of 25 and 34 watches 27 and one-half hours of television, each and every week. That's more than one *day*. But if you find that figure shocking, consider this – it goes up as we age. By the time we reach the 35 – 44 brackets, we're in for 33 hours and 40 minutes. After 45, the figure rises again to almost 44 hours per week.

That is one helluva lot of time. Some couples even watch television in different rooms, exacerbating the damaging effect this modern habit can have by adding physical isolation.

I'm going to assume that most of you are in the median group (35 – 44). Can we agree that you're still young and healthy (for the most part) and sexually robust? Can we agree you're still interested in regular sex with your partner, because you're reading this book? Then maybe it's time to kick your sex-undermining little friend out of the house, for good. We did it and we're glad. We spend our time on other things, now, including sex. Sex isn't just for Saturday night at our house (although it's part of the weekend fun). Because we have exiled the insidious influence of television from our home, we are healthier, more engaged with each and happier, all around. We have time, because we've made it our bitch by making one simple change in our lives.

Back to that "roommate" thing

OK. I know sweatpants are comfortable. The thing is that if they become your home uniform, then you have effectively "de-sexified" yourself. This is true whether you are a man or a woman. Throw those things away. I mean it. My love became a bit too attached to her pair of well-worn sweats. I got to the point at which I wondered if she had lost all her other clothes, except those she wore to work. So I asked her:

"Did something happen to your other clothes?"

"No," she answered, regarding me with wide, curious eyes. "Why are you asking me that?"

As gently as possible, I asked her where the silk lounging pajamas I'd brought her from the last convention I'd attended. I told her how sexy I thought she'd look in them and asked why she never wore them.

"Those are for special occasions, honey!" She giggled, coyly.

"Every day is a special occasion, where you're concerned." I said, smiling sweetly.

Without telling her she looked like a homeless person, or dumpy, I made it clear that the sweatpants were not doing it for me; that I wanted to enjoy her glory swaddled in something perhaps more enticing than those frigging sweats. I had planned for the occasion, thought about what I intended to say and how I intended to say it, beforehand. I'd also tidied up my own appearance, in preparation. Sauce. Goose. Gander. Women are visual, too, fellas. They like to see the man they originally fell in love with, occasionally.

Chapter 4 Explore Him/Her Body

The Female Body

Many women are faced with societal pressures and social conditioning that can easily prevent them from connecting their sexual energy and engaging in sexual acts and behaviors solely for the purpose of fulfilling their own desires, rather than as an obligation to fulfill those of their partners. When a woman begins to understand that her sexuality and sexual nature are beautiful, powerful and positive, she can enjoy being sexually stimulated and nurtured by her lover. Helping her to realize her own orgasmic capacity and also be able to expand it, is one of the goals and outcomes of Tantric sex, and this chapter will explore Tantric methods and practices by which women can both be pleased by their partners.

The Yoni (Vagina)

"Yoni" (pronounced YO-nee) is the Sanskrit word for the vagina. The vagina is sacred in Tantra, and thus must be treated with the utmost care and respect. The Yoni massage is a sensuous technique that both emotionally and spiritually brings partners closer together, building trust and intimacy along the way.

How to Give a Tantric Yoni Massage

While the Yoni massage is definitely stimulating, remember that the main purpose is to relax both partners and encourage emotions to rise to the surface. Women may experience a variety of sensations and feelings during this massage ranging from lust to anger, to excitement, or indifference and all of this is a good thing! Remember, during the Yoni massage, there are no boundaries, as there is no focus on achieving any desired outcome other than to feel, observe, connect, and experience. As your skills improve and you move toward mastery of the Yoni massage, your understanding of female sexuality will deepen and your sex life as a whole will be much improved.

Breathing is a Tantric foreplay activity that assists in building emotional and spiritual bonds between lovers. Prior to beginning the Yoni massage, first spend some time increasing awareness of each other's' essence and presence by gazing into each other's eyes, embracing, and engaging in deep, synchronized breathing. The giver of the upcoming massage should take the lead in the breathing exercise, but both the giver and receiver should remain focused and relaxed during the entire activity. Should the receiver begin to stop, pause or take more shallow breaths, the giver should gently remind her of the pace and depth that she should be striving to meet.

When both parties feel sufficiently relaxed, comfortable and connected, the receiver should lie on her back with a pillow beneath her neck for comfort, and another underneath her hips, elevating her pelvis. She pulls her legs up by bending her knees with her feet flat on the bed or floor, and opens her legs, exposing her Yoni, while the giver sits cross-legged in between her open legs, on a pillow or cushion if desired.

The giver should begin by massaging other parts of her body, encouraging relaxation. Firmly and gently massage her arms, breasts, stomach, hips, and thighs before moving inward to her pelvic region. Continue by massaging her pubic bone, working your way to the inner thigh. Repeat this action, at least nine times, then use the right hand to apply a lubricant or oil to the top or mound of the Yoni, making sure that enough is poured so that the outer lips and outside of the Yoni are covered.

Rub the lubricant on the outer lips several times, as she will find this highly erotic and pleasurable. With the thumb and index finger of each hand, apply light pressure and squeeze each of her Yoni lips, sliding your oiled fingers up and down the entire length of each one. Once the outer lips are complete, repeat the process with each inner lip, paying close attention to her preferences, altering the pressure and speed according to her physical and audible cues.

The next step, clitoral stimulation, is optional and may or may not be possible, depending on her level of sensitivity to clitoral stimulation. You will have to pay close attention to her cues and expressed desires before going too far into clitoral stimulation, but if this is something that she enjoys, begin by stroking her clitoris in a gentle, circular motion. Next, while squeezing her clitoris between your thumb and index finger, rotate your hand until your wrist faces upward, carefully and slowly insert your middle finger into her Yoni, and explore the inside of her with your finger. Take your time and enjoy the way she feels. With varying degrees of speed and depth, feel up, down, right and left until you reach her "sacred spot" -- her G-spot.

Continue with the massage switching up the intensity, speed and direction. Maintain the connectivity of deep breathing and looking into each other's' eyes. At this point, she may experience waves of powerful emotion, begin to shiver, shake and cry, but no matter what, keep breathing, keep encouraging her to breathe, and remain gentle. If she does reach orgasm, ask her if she would like you to continue. At this point, if you continue, she will likely have multiple orgasms in a row, each more intense than the last. In Tantra, this exciting experience is known as "riding the wave", and many women -- even those who have never experienced orgasm before -- can learn to become multi-orgasmic when the Tantric Yoni Massage is correctly performed by a gentle, patient partner.

Your job is to keep massaging and enjoying the moment until she assures you that she is ready to stop. At that time, allow her to relish the moment and enjoy the afterglow of the powerful orgasms you have given her while you enjoy the satisfaction of pleasing your woman and creating a special moment together.

The Clitoris

The clitoris is positioned in between the labia above the vagina. It consists of two parts -- the rounded glans and the longer shaft -- which is covered by a "hood" of skin, the clitoral hood. While most, if not all, women can reach orgasm from clitoral stimulation, as stated earlier in this book, some women are too sensitive in this area so it is always a good idea to check with the woman to see how much clitoral stimulation works for her. Regardless, it is important to make sure that you use enough lubrication when venturing to manipulate any woman's clitoris. You'll never want to touch that extremely sensitive area without adequate lubrication.

How to Give a Tantric Clitoral Massage

The purpose of the Tantric clitoral massage is to make the woman's clitoris the center of attention. This massage can be given alone, as part of a Yoni massage, part of the G-spot massage (which will be covered in the next section), or part of a standard erotic massage.

If the Tantric clitoral massage is not an extension of another session where you have already set the mood, make sure to create a warming, inviting, special ambiance where your partner will feel relaxed and open. Either ask her to undress, or slowly undress her yourself, and request that she lie face down once she is fully nude. Give her a full body massage, starting on her back working your way from neck to toe. After several minutes, turn her over, and then work your back up from her feet to her shoulders and neck.

Avoid massaging her breasts or genitalia for the time being to tease her and build momentum. The goal here is to heighten her senses, keep her guessing, and to invite her to expect the unexpected.

After you have massaged every inch of her body except for her genitalia and are ready to begin the clitoral massage, gently touch either of her knees, sliding your hand up her inner thigh, continuing up to her vulva. Depending on the size and sensitivity of her clitoris, you will be massaging it using between one and three fingers. As a rule:

    a. If you can feel her clitoral shaft with your fingers, use your thumb and index finger (2 fingers).

    b. If her clitoris is larger and more prominent, you can use your thumb, index finger, and middle finger (3 fingers).

    c. On the contrary, if her clitoris is small and hidden, use either the tip of your index finger or your thumb (1 finger).

If you are only using one finger, place either the tip of your finger or your thumb atop her clitoris, move the skin underneath your finger either around in tiny circles or back and forth. Even if her clitoris is small and hidden, you should be able to feel it hardening and becoming more erect as she becomes more aroused.

If you are using more than one finger, lightly grasp the shaft with your thumb and index finger while gently sliding the tissue surrounding her clitoris back and forth in order to determine clitoral shape and firmness. It is important to determine how much the tissue around her clitoris slides around because you do not want to apply too much pressure. You want to avoid grasping the glans directly if possible, but the goal here is for the hood to slide back and forth as you manipulate the shaft, which will indirectly stimulate her glans.

Place your thumb and forefinger around the hood, lightly pinch the clitoris and gently roll it around between your fingers. Pull the hood up so that the clitoris is exposed, and blow on it. Use a heavily lubricated fingertip to gently tease it in different directions -- up, down, left, right, or in circles -- and pay attention to what she responds to best. This action will bring blood to the surface and charge her nerve endings.

If she is enjoying herself, continue in a steady rhythm. As her level of arousal increases, you can experiment with increasing pressure, but always remember to be gentle. You can vary the speed of your strokes from very slow and methodic in the beginning, making them increasingly faster as she nears orgasm.

Once she reaches orgasm, move your fingers away from her clitoris and to her labia. Maintain physical contact as she recovers from her orgasmic high. Once she has recovered you can either start over again or stop, but please never stop the massage abruptly unless she expresses discomfort. In this case, shift your focus to her vulva or other less sensitive areas in her pelvic region for a few minutes until she is ready to proceed.

Although she may orgasm very quickly and easily, it may take some time for both of you to get comfortable with this technique. The best way to figure out how to give and receive the Tantric clitoral massage is through keeping open minds and gaining experience through practicing together, which can be a great bonding experience.

The Breasts: How to Give a Tantric Breast Massage

The Tantric breast massage is a special ritual that allows a woman to receive sensual energy from her partner. Massaging the breasts makes them firmer and healthier while maintaining the hormonal balance within a woman's body. The Tantric breast massage is a way for one to please, heal and become more intimate with their partner, as the breasts need to be loved and honored first before other elements of her body will become free to open.

Breast tissue is delicate, but with proper technique and moderate pressure, a Tantric breast massage can be simple and safe. Make sure that the woman is in a warm, safe space before beginning, and verbally communicate to her that the massage is purely for her enjoyment and that she need not wonder about giving you pleasure at all.

Before beginning the massage, place one hand on her heart and the other on her Yoni and visualize energy moving from your heart into your hands and toward her heart and Yoni. This visualization is connection and healing and an important part of this Tantric massage session.

To avoid friction, apply massage oil onto the breast in circular motions going from the center of the chest into the underarm region. Caress her breasts slowly and gently, brushing the palms of your hands over the entire breast. Get into a rhythm, repeat your moves, at least twenty times at a consistent pace and pressure. First, try going clockwise on both breasts. Then try the following move:

1. Place your palm over her entire breast with the nipple in the center.
2. Fan your fingers out, mimicking a wheel spoke.
3. Slowly bring your fingers in toward the nipple.
4. Finish with a slight (or firmer if you so desire) pinch.
5. Repeat.

After the above technique is applied, the second step is to gently knead the fully covered breasts by lifting them from the chest, pressing delicately. Alternating breasts one after the other, methodically twist and wring each one in rhythmic fashion, at least twenty times.

The third step is to gently attempt to "scoop" the flesh with the flat of the fingertips; first clockwise, then counterclockwise.

Fourth, you will directly massage the nipples. Place both thumbs on opposite sides of the nipple of one breast, starting at the outside edge of her areola (the dark, flat circle surrounding her actual nipple). Slowly bring your thumbs together, squeezing the nipple between the thumbs, then pull outwards toward you. Do this until a complete circle is made around her nipple, adjusting the pressure based on her reaction. Repeat on the other breast.

Finally, during the "cooling down" phase of the massage, you will stroke and smooth her skin. Take the fingertips of both hands toward the center of one breast and radiate them from the center outward toward the side. Do this, at least ten times, and then repeat on the other breast.

The breast massage ends the same way it began, with one hand on her heart and the other on her

Yoni, visualizing warm energy moving from your heart into your hands and down into her heart and Yoni. Breathe deeply and slowly together for several minutes, and then allow her to rest.

While the primary purpose of the Tantric breast massage is to please the receiver, it is enjoyable for the giver too. It is not only emotionally and physically healing, but it provides relaxation and a sensuous form of foreplay. It can be done alone or as the introduction to other Tantric massages such as the Yoni massage, clitoral massage, or G-spot massage.

The G-Spot

The G-spot (Grafenberg spot) is a tiny lima-bean shaped region located on the front (tummy-side) wall of the Yoni, two to three inches beneath the pubic bone. This area is different in texture than the rest of the Yoni, in that it is spongier and coarse. G-spot stimulation causes intense orgasmic feelings that are greater than in a normal sexual response.

How to Give a Tantric G-Spot Massage

In Tantra, the G-spot is known to store creative sexual energy, but also has another side; it stores sexual or emotional pain as well. Therefore, the G-spot massage, when performed correctly, can be healing as it can remove blocks to sexual pleasure, replacing them with positive sensations.

Once the receiver of the massage is undressed and lying face down, begin by giving her a ten-minute full-body massage. Once she is fully relaxed, ask her politely if you may massage her more intimately. If she obliges, gently massage her pubic area including the lips of her Yoni with high-quality lubricant.

Upon arousal, whisper in her ear that you are going to put your fingers inside of her. Lubricate your first two fingers well, insert them as far into her Yoni as is comfortable for her, and move them in even circles all around. Keep in mind that consistent, firm pressure along the entire length of the vaginal walls normally feels best, but you'll have to take her physical and audible cues as guides, as every woman is unique in her preferences. As a tip: pressing the palm of your other hand on the top of her pelvis can be very "grounding" for her.

Envision the G-spot as a clock. Spend a little bit of time with your fingers at each position of the clock. Pay attention to which "hours" feel best, which are numb, which may be painful, and which trigger some emotional reaction. If you find a great spot, press gently and hold. If any strong emotions arise such as anger, sadness or laughter, gently encourage her to describe anything she feels or "sees". Allow the energy to discharge, for this release of energy is healing and makes her sexual energy more available.

As the massage develops, begin to concentrate on pleasing her rather than on the numb or painful places. Another great way to stimulate the G-spot is by using the "press-and-release" technique:

1. Hook your fingers, pulling the G-spot upward.

2. Rhythmically press and release.

When the G-spot massage is finished, tell her that you are going to remove your fingers. As you gently slide your fingers out of her, press the mound of her vagina with your free hand, thus sealing the end of the Tantric G-spot Yoni healing process.

As a word of caution, it is important not to have any expectations regarding the outcome of this massage. Results may not be immediately visible and it may take a few tries before any emotions arise. In the meantime, take pleasure in becoming more familiar with your partner's Yoni and building a stronger bond between the two of you.

G-Spot Orgasms

Two conditions must be met to stimulate the G-spot. First, the woman must be aroused and secondly, pressure must be applied on the upper vaginal wall. Blood rushes to the G-spot similarly to how it does to the clitoris when a woman is sufficiently aroused, thus, any sexual position which places pressure on the area leads to greater chances of the woman experiencing the orgasm.

The Male Body

The Lingam (Penis)

"Lingam" is the Sanskrit word for the penis and is literally translated to mean "wand of light". In

Tantra, the Lingam is viewed with respect and honored as a wand of light that channels energy and pleasure. Orgasm may offer a pleasant side-effect to receipt of a Lingam massage, but it is never the goal. The goal is to massage the organ, encouraging a man to relax and surrender to a deeper form of pleasure that he may not be used to.

Men must learn to relax and receive pleasure that is not goal (orgasm) oriented, as is common with traditional sexual expectation.

Taoist belief holds that the Lingam has reflex points similar to those in the feet or hands which when stimulated properly can affect the whole organ, allowing the massage to be both healing and sexual simultaneously. Applying pressure to different pressure points in the Lingam disperses energy to the entire body, leading to a wave-like experience of pleasure. This energy is dispersed all over the body, and then is built upon. In this fashion, men are able to experience full-body orgasms, and this wave of pleasure can last for a much longer time than a regular orgasm.

How to Give a Tantric Lingam Massage

Prepare a quiet dim space with a bed, futon, or a blanket and pillows on the floor. Make sure that the temperature is slightly warmer than normal, as you will both be nude. Lighting candles is an excellent idea both for lighting and temperature regulation. Your high-quality oils and lubricants should be within reach. Using spill-resistant bottles and plastic instead of glass is advised. And most of all make sure that you have a few hours of uninterrupted time so that you won't feel rushed.

Begin by standing or sitting face-to-face, and breathe deeply together. Touch each other by embracing or holding hands while looking into each other's eyes, breathing rhythmically from the belly. If he begins to hold his breath or lose focus, position one hand on his lower belly, and encourage him to breathe from that place and "fill his belly" with breath.

Have him lie face down and give him a full-body massage for at least ten minutes. Request that he turn over, and then continue his massage. Advance the massage toward the inner thighs and pelvis until his entire body is relaxed.

As a show of respect for his male power, ask for permission to touch his Lingam. If he is familiar with Tantric terminology, ask "May I touch your Wand of Light"? Otherwise asking "May I touch your Lingam?" or "May I touch your penis?" will suffice. If he obliges, cover his Lingam and testicles with the oil or lubricant. Rub the solution into his skin, starting at the top of his inner thighs, moving into the crease where his legs meet the pelvis. Release tension as you work along the connecting tissue, bone and muscles using slow, steady motions.

Continue by massaging above the Lingam on the pubic bone. Place one hand over this area, feeling the bone beneath the muscle. Slowly work your way down to the scrotum, very gently pulling on his testicles. It is important to pay attention to his physical and audible cues, as well as encourage him to let you know what feels right to him, as some men are averse to testicular pressure, while others very much enjoy stronger handling. Begin gently and slowly build pressure until you find the perfect amount.

Finally, slowly place one hand on the Lingam with your right hand. As you massage the shaft, squeeze the Lingam at the very bottom with your right hand, pull up, and slide completely off. Then alternate hands. Repeat this motion with each hand several times, and then switch direction -- slide alternating hands from the top back down to the base.

Take the Lingam between both hands and rub your hands together quickly as if attempting to start a fire. Hold the Lingam by the head and gently shake back and forth. Massage the head, cupping it in your palm and turning your wrist as if juicing a lemon.

If at any time he seems close to ejaculation, slow your movements and let him "cool down" before continuing. If he is close but not past the point of no return, you may be able to delay ejaculation by squeezing the tip of the Lingam between the thumb and forefinger very firmly and holding it for about thirty seconds, encouraging him to take deep breaths the entire time.

If you are successfully able to hold back his orgasm six times, tons of sexual energy will be stored. He can then retain and circulate this energy throughout his body, or choose to release. If he does choose to ejaculate, a much more intense orgasm than usual will be experienced. Remind him to take deep, controlled breaths as he ejaculates. Once the massage is complete, tell him that you will now remove your hands and allow him time to relax and enjoy the mind-blowing pleasure he has received.

The Testicles

Testicle massages can infuse the testicles with blood and clear out any blockages. Massaging the testicles on a regular basis can improve erections, ejaculation volume, and sperm count. The massage even has the potential to increase testicular size, making them fuller-feeling, lower-hanging, and more sensitive.

How to Give a Tantric Testicle Massage

Testicles are the most sensitive part of most men's' bodies, as such, many women fear massaging the area for fear of causing pain. The irony behind this is that it is exactly this sensitivity that incites pleasure once the area is stroked. The testicles can be one of the most erogenous spots on his body if stimulated properly, and a good testicle massage can be an outstanding experience for a man if a lover is doing it.

Once a safe, warm, ambient place is set and your man is comfortable and ready, here are eight steps that you can try to give a pleasing Tantric testicle massage:

1. Trace circles around the base of the penis where the shaft is attached to the scrotum.

2. Very lightly pinch the scrotal skin, gently rolling the skin between your fingers, and monitor his response.

3. Very lightly run your fingernails across the skin of his scrotum, paying close attention to his reaction. Some men absolutely love this sensation while others become nervous. If he likes it, continue. If not, stop.

4. With a firm grip, wrap your hands around his penis. Slide one hand up over the head and the other down across the

testicles. This motion makes the penis feel big, expanding the sensation.

5. Cup the testicles and give them a gentle squeeze. Monitor his reaction, making sure that you aren't squeezing too hard.

6. Placing your hand at the bottom of the testicles, run your fingers from the bottom of the scrotum all the way up to the head of the penis in one smooth motion.

7. Hold the penis up, exposing the testicles, and tap them lightly with your middle finger.

8. Hold the penis and testicles in between the thumb and forefinger of one hand. Pull them both forward with your hand. Do this at least ten times in each direction -- up, down, left, and right.

Chapter 5 How to Give an Erotic Massage to Help Increase Intimacy

There are many different ways to give a Tantric massage and in time you will learn how to develop your OWN massage techniques suited to you and your partner. However, if you are confused as to how to begin, here is a guide, or rather two, on how to give your partner a sensual, Tantric massage:

Before you attempt how to learn to give a tantric massage, you have to take care of the ingredients you will be using. Learn them, put them together in the right combination and you will see your partner being very happy indeed. A Tantric massage delivered well and good can be one of the greatest doorways to passion.

Set the Mood

This is an extremely important part of tantric massage. This massage is supposed to be sexy and that will not be possible unless you are both into it. The best way to get into a situation is by setting the atmosphere or the mood of the room at a level of ease at which you are both able to indulge and lose yourself.

There are many ways you can set the mood. Try to alter the lighting by making it dim but not too dark. This provides a comfortable ambiance and will help your partner believe that their body looks sexy in the semi-darkness. Next, prepare the station. You will do this according to the type of massage you will be attempting to give. If it is a simple head or shoulder massage, you only need a chair. Otherwise it would be nice to prepare a stable surface such as a table or even the floor. Just remember that the surface needs to be firm enough for them to lie down so you can work your magic.

Music

This is an essential part of setting the correct mood for the massage. Note that in these situations, rough music such as heavy metal won't work. Choose something according to what your goal is. Sometimes you might want to give a massage to get them in the mood for sex and others you might want them to relax and drift off to sleep. Choose accordingly. If you are going for sex, choose something like intimate soul music. If you are going for relaxation, choose soft blues or nature sounds. Running water is especially soothing to help someone drift off.

The Oil

This is the vital ingredient for your massage. Consider this your turkey to your thanksgiving dinner. There are several different oils you can use, such as avocado, jojoba and grape seed oil. Experiment with a few and find what you like or what suits your partner the best. These oils are all usually available at health food stores, spa shops or skincare stores. You can even buy pre-blended massage oils that contain two or more oils. Make sure to buy any oil that helps your hands glide easily without chafing your partner's skin. Remember, comfort is the most important part of the whole massage.

Try and buy organic oil in small quantities and then store it in a cool and dry place.

Tantric Massage Techniques

This part will consist of two separate methods, one that will help you massage a female body and the other that caters to a male body's needs of the same. Fundamentally, both bodies are more or less the same but their treatment is somewhat different. Hence, here is the correct way to massage a female body:

Of course massages vary from type to type but one of the best tantric massages is the full body massage because it helps a person to relax under your touch and increases intimacy between you both.

Try and practice the techniques that are about to be relayed to you on your own body so that you know that you aren't being too hard on your recipient as well. Your thigh should be perfect to practice on.

Shiatsu

This is one of the easiest and most commonly used massage techniques in Japan. If you have received a massage with someone rubbing the knots under your skin out using their thumbs or elbows, you have had the shiatsu style massage treatment.

The technique involves placing your fingers or hands upon a particular place on her body. Apply gentle pressure and then move your hand or finger in a circular motion. The best spot for using this technique is the upper back, so use it to loosen up the knots in that area. Just make sure that you don't compress so hard that you cause her pain!

You might have seen experienced massage therapists applying pressure by using their elbows. However, this is an advanced technique that you should avoid unless you have real experience or are a licensed masseuse.

Compression

Compression is another popular method for massage. In order to perform a compression massage, you must apply pressure to one area of your partners' body. This will increase the flow of blood to this area and remove tension and rigidity from the muscle. This massage is much like a warm-up for the more intense styles of massage such as shiatsu. If you are extremely tense, don't go for shiatsu immediately because its intensity might injure you. Instead, have your partner give you a compression massage, it will boost blood flow and loosen up your muscles for shiatsu.

Stroking

The name of this massage is very descriptive. Stroking massages are very different from compression or shiatsu massages in that applying concentrated pressure does not perform them. Instead, this massage involves sliding your hands across parts of her body such as her thighs or back. It is a very stimulating form of massage and become extremely erotic if you do it right. It is also minimal in its intensity and a lot easier to do than compression or shiatsu massages.

Friction

This is a high-level technique that can be applied to the more bonier parts of your partners body such as her hands or feet. In this technique, you do not need to use oils. Instead, you must use your dry hands to generate heat via friction. The strokes must be firm but no hard, as compression is not required. In fact, compression would an impediment to the speed at which your hand is traveling across her body. This type of massage is in many ways a more advanced technique than stroking.

Kneading

This massage is amazing for reaching into deeper parts of her muscles and is especially good for relieving tension from the fleshy areas such as the buttocks. Be very gentle because you do not want to harm her. Do not perform this massage on her stomach because that will make her feel uncomfortable.

If you have ever baked bread before, you will realize that this massage is similar to kneading bread. To knead the muscles, take hold of the muscle and give it a slight dig with your fingers whilst raising the tissue with your thumbs. Do not lift too high because that will hurt. First, you will press your palm into their muscles, and then you will squeeze their muscles slightly and then give a gentle lift with your thumb. Try it gently on your thigh and use the same gentle motions on her skin. This massage is also good for her shoulders especially if you sense a tension in them. Remember to give her a little Shiatsu first, however, since directly kneading an already tense shoulder or neck muscle can be quite painful.

These massages are excellent if you combine them. Mixing up shiatsu, oil massage, compression, stroking and friction can be a great way to keep things interesting. Remember, doing the same thing over and over again will get boring for the both of you and will stop being effective after a little while, so apply different massage techniques to different parts of the body and your lover will be in heaven by the time you are done.

Tantric Massage for Males

The tantric massage for a man will be different than the normal erotic massage. Remember that a man might be more wary of a massage than a female though he may not show it. Put your partner at ease before you initiate this massage because you will be touching them in a way that might seem too intimate to their masculinity, hence be prepared to be gentle without seeming like you are patronizing them.

If you wish to massage your partner's penis, it is highly recommended that you use some kind of oil to make it easier to rub. Massaging a dry penis can result in chafing and is usually not nearly as enjoyable as a massage that is performed with oil.

Using oil in this manner will also prevent you from potentially injuring your partner during the act of massaging.

A good massage that involves tantric practice would require the use of both of your hands. This is because you have several areas that you would ideally have to stimulate, and stimulating at least two areas at the same time will greatly boost the amount of arousal that your partner experiences.

Try to stroke his penis up and down whilst simultaneously massaging his testicles. His testicles are extremely sensitive, which means that if you gently stimulate them he is going to feel a ticklish and warm sensation within his penis. This will make him feel as though he is perpetually about to have an orgasm throughout your massage!

Chapter 6 Unlocking Intimate Capacity Through Synergy

The best lovemaking experiences come when you and your partner are moving and flowing in harmony with one another. Perhaps you have experienced this for yourself. What is the best sexual experience you've ever had? No matter what "type" of sex you had or with whom, it is likely that you and your partner were embodying the same energy and matching one another's passion. Whether you had rough sex, slow sex, sleepy sex, or spontaneous sex, the best sex comes from a perfect synergy between you and your partner.

The unfortunate thing is that we don't always know how to create this synergy; it just happens. The right environment, the right mood, the right time of day, and some other accidental factors often contribute to our most mind-blowing sex.

The heart of the Tantric sex practice is learning how to intentionally create the right elements to have the deep, intense, mind-blowing sex that everyone craves. In the last chapter, we learned how to set up one's physical environment to stimulate the senses and nurture deep intimacy. Now we will look at the internal factors that contribute to amazing, long-lasting, and profoundly fulfilling sex.

What is Energy?

Perhaps the most important aspect of Tantric practice is the energy that you and your partner bring into the experience. Without the right energy, all your setup and foreplay won't be nearly as effective in contributing to the overall Tantric experience. Setup and foreplay can certainly aid you in establishing the best energy for sex, but to get it just right, more intentional energy work is needed. True Tantra is much more about energy than about sex, wherein the focus is on merging the energies within yourself and then merging your united energy with that of your partner.

So, what is energy? Energy is the animating force behind all of the creation. It is what causes the movement of atoms, the formation of matter, and the evolution of life. Beyond the realm of the physical, energy is what composes the soul or spirit. It is what connects us to the center of divine creation itself.

When we talk about our energy, we are in part talking about the electromagnetic field that surrounds all bodies and the electric force within that animates our bodily functions. However, our energy is also composed of the spirit within our bodies, which is also made of energy.

Energy can take different forms. You may hear people talk about "good" and "bad" energy, or "positive" and "negative" energy. What they mean by this is that the emotions and intentions of which others "send out" their energy. When someone performs an action with kind and loving intentions, people say that they have "good" energy, whereas when someone does or says something that is fueled by anger or is meant to be hurtful, we say they have "bad" energy.

When we talk about people "sending" energy, we are discussing the actions, emotions, thoughts, and intentions that they manifest. While raw energy is essentially neutral, our thoughts and emotions can "bend" or "tint" our energy to match the tone of those thoughts and emotions. Others can pick up on our energy and interpret our intentions based on what they perceive. Hence, when people say that they will send us "good vibes" or "healing energy," what they mean is that they will have loving and positive thoughts about us and wish us well.

Energy is a complex force that can be used and interpreted in many ways. Since energy is the raw force behind all of the creation, we use energy in its purest expression when we create. We often do this unconsciously, allowing our reactive natures to determine what energy we put out into the world. However, when we start to become aware of our own energy and watch our thoughts and actions more carefully, we gain the power to choose the energy that we send into the world, which, in turn, determines what energy we are most likely to receive from others.

How to Recognize Energy

To reach a full understanding of what energy is and how to recognize and control it, you can start to practice in two different ways. First, you will learn how to recognize the electromagnetic field around your own body and that of your partner. From there, you will start to work with recognizing the energy around you as it manifests from others' thoughts, emotions, and intentions.

Learning to recognize your electromagnetic field is very simple, but it will take practice to get good at it. To begin, rub your hands together vigorously. You will start to feel the heat generated between your palms as the friction warms your skin. After a few moments, slowly begin to pull your hands apart, holding them just far enough apart that the skin of your palms is no longer touching. You will continue to feel the heat you generated by rubbing your hands together, as well as a slight tingling sensation.

Slowly begin to pull your hands further apart until they are about a half-inch away from one another. If you can still feel the warm, tingling sensation of your electromagnetic field, then you can move your hands to an inch apart. If you lose the feeling, move your hands closer together and start over.

Continue the exercise by pulling your hands further and further apart. If at any point you lose the tingling sensation, bring them closer together and move slowly apart again. Feel free to start over as many times as you need. The goal is to be able to sense the energy between your hands even when they are a foot apart or more. Advanced energy practitioners learn to shape and move energy for healing, but that is another line of study beyond what we will learn with Tantra.

You can begin to move your energy awareness to the rest of your body with another simple exercise. Bring your attention to one of your forearms, focusing as much as you can on the surface of your skin. When you are fully aware of your forearm, pull your attention to a quarter of an inch above your arm. If you can feel a sensation at that distance, you have found your energy field. If not, return your focus to your skin and begin again.

Like the hand exercise, you will continue to pull your focus farther and farther away from the surface of your skin. If at any point you lose your sense of your electromagnetic field, go back and begin again. Researchers have found that our energy fields extend an average of 10-15 feet beyond our physical bodies, so you can take this practice quite far before you will reach the edge of your energy field.

If understanding and sensing our own energy is difficult, learning to sense the energy of others is a much more complex matter. Knowing the energy of the people around us comes from a number of factors. Most of us begin to learn to recognize others' moods and reactions from their body language, the tone of voice, and facial expressions at a very young age. This innate sense certainly plays a role in our ability to sense the energy of others, though true energy awareness goes much further than that.

As you grow your awareness of your own energy field, you will slowly begin to feel when other people's energy fields collide with your own. If the sensation is pleasant or neutral, then you know that those people have "positive" or "neutral" energy that is in harmony with your own. If the feeling makes you uncomfortable, then that person likely has "bad" energy.

Another major part of learning to read others' energy is by developing your intuition. We can often tell what others are thinking or feeling in spite of their physical cues, especially our loved ones. We can't always explain these feelings; we just "know." This knowing, otherwise commonly referred to as a "gut feeling," is our intuition.

Accepting and trusting your intuition is the first step in developing it. The easiest way to validate your intuition is to practice with your loved ones. If you feel that you are picking up on emotions beneath the surface when talking to a friend or family member, ask them if anything else is going on. People often acknowledge their true emotions when prompted, even when they feel the need to keep them hidden in general.

You'll encounter plenty of other opportunities to develop your intuition as you go through life. Sometimes you'll have an intuition to drive or walk one way instead of another or to choose one line at the bank or grocery store over the others. Learn to follow these feelings and great things will very often follow a pleasant conversation, an interesting find, or even the avoidance of some sort of accident. Your intuition is a powerful part of yourself that can aid you in many aspects of life, and it introduces an interesting element in the sexual experience for those who work to develop it.

Using Energy to Deepen Sexual Pleasure

Cultivating an awareness of your energy and your partner's will enable you to harmonize and channel your energies to create a smooth flow through your sexual experience. When both participants focus their intentions on creating a loving, open, and sensual, sexual encounter, the results can be astounding.

The first step to synchronizing your energy with your partner is to communicate openly about what kind of experience you both wish to have. If both partners want a different kind of sexual encounter, it is best to compromise so that both feel their needs are met. It is better to speak openly about what you want and what makes you uncomfortable rather than to see your desires collide mid-experience.

When you have agreed upon the type of sexual experience you both want, you and your partner can spend a few minutes setting your mutual intentions at the beginning of your ritual. Including intentions such as, "To have a healthy and nurturing experience together," "To achieve great emotional and sexual healing together," "To give each other the maximum amount of pleasure possible in an open and safe environment," or "To deepen our bond and create an experience that will make us feel closer to one another," are all appropriate intentions.

When establishing the energy for your sexual experience, it is crucial that both partners agree to only engage in sex if it is mutually wanted. Sometimes we get so busy in our lives that we need to schedule our intimacy to fit around our other obligations. However, when the time and day come, we might be too tired or stressed to feel like engaging sexually. Often, an argument or misunderstanding will create tension with our partners and we might not feel like sex is the best thing to do while there is discomfort between us.

If these situations should arise, it has to be okay for you to honor one another's feelings and not pressure each other into sex. You could agree to have a non-sexual Tantric session, where you will just massage and pamper one another, or you could talk through your issues or enjoy some other healing activity together. If both people are not completely on board with having sex, it is best not to compromise the integrity of your energy by trying to push forward.

However, if both people are completely ready and willing, you can harmonize your energies for the sexual experience by both showing up in a happy and loving mood. Allow yourself to feel all the love, compassion, and devotion to your partner at the start of your ritual. By opening the Tantric session with the right energy, you will ensure that you will both have the best sexual experience possible.

The Masculine and Feminine Aspects of the Self

Many of us are familiar with the concept of duality: for every state, there is an opposite. For every light, a dark; for every night, a day; for every hot, a cold; for every negative, a positive. The masculine and feminine are fundamental aspects of dual nature that are present in all of the existence. However, whereas philosophies of duality hold that these polar opposites usually remain separate, even when they meet, in Tantric philosophy, all opposites merge into one.

Everyone, whether men, women, or non-binary individuals, hold both masculine and feminine aspects within their beings. The masculine and feminine have less to do with one's gender than within the traits that one embodies. Some people have more masculine traits, while others have more feminine—and then there are those who have a nearly equal balance of both.

The masculine is assertive, active, direct, hard, linear, and focused. It is also associated with the aspects of light, heat, dry, and positive. The feminine, on the other hand, is passive, still, indirect, soft, circular, and abstract. It is associated with the aspects of dark, cold, wet, and negative. Whereas the masculine is the penetrating force, the feminine is receptive. The masculine bestows the seed of creation, while the feminine provides the ground for the seed to grow. The masculine is protective while the feminine is nurturing.

While everyone has the capacity for all these traits, some people embody more from one side of the spectrum than the other. When this happens, an imbalance might be present, and it is time to work on restoring harmony between the different aspects of the self.

How to Balance and Unify Your Masculine and Feminine

You may have observed many of these traits within yourself. Certain situations may evoke your more masculine traits, while others evoke your feminine. Many people naturally lean more one way than the other, usually in the direction of their physical gender. However, when an extreme imbalance is present, the effects can be harmful to the individual and those in their lives.

When there is an imbalance of masculine energy, people often become overly aggressive, confrontational, and hostile. The shadow side of the masculine is its tendency to pick fights and engage in ego battles. People with too much masculine energy can be egotistical and narcissistic, often bullying others into getting their way and refusing to listen to others. At its worst, the shadow masculine can be abusive and controlling.

A feminine imbalance, on the other hand, can lead individuals to be overly passive. These people refuse to assert their needs, to stand up for themselves, or to make things happen in their lives. They can be sensitive to the point that they can barely function, and they may listen to what others need more than working to meet their own needs. They can be scattered, unfocused, and messy. The worst of the shadow feminine is a tendency towards victimhood and martyrdom.

Balancing the masculine and the feminine is a necessary process that takes time and effort. When both aspects of the self are in balance, however, the individual can experience peace, harmony, and health within.

The first step to creating balance is to recognize where there are imbalances. Did either of the above descriptions resonate with you? When you identify which areas you need to balance out, then you can begin to cultivate aspects of the other energy.

For instance, if you are imbalanced in the direction of the masculine, you may be overly aggressive and independent, refusing to accept help from others, even when you need it the most. To correct this imbalance, you'll have to cultivate your feminine traits of patience, cooperation, and receptivity to allow yourself to slow down and include others in your endeavors.

On the other hand, if you have a feminine imbalance, you might be too dependent on others, too passive, and unable to get things done on your own. In this case, you would have to cultivate the masculine traits of independence and assertiveness to push through your obstacles and do what needs to be done.

Once your masculine and feminine energies are balanced, then you can begin to work on unifying them. Inner union comes when you accept all aspects of yourself and allow them to manifest in your life naturally. This could be particularly difficult for some who have learned that embodying one type of energy is "dangerous." For instance, people with a masculine imbalance may have learned at an early age that showing emotion and becoming vulnerable will only get them hurt, so they have become overly defensive and emotionally unavailable to compensate. Others may have been punished earlier on for asserting themselves and decided that being overly passive was a safer course of action.

As an adult, you have the power to write a new story for yourself and to build a life that makes it safe for you to embrace and embody all parts of yourself. It is only through full acceptance that you can unify your aspects within. Once you are whole, you can bring your wholeness forward in your lovemaking practices.

Enhancing Your Lovemaking with Masculine and Feminine Energy

Tantric sex holds the potential for significant healing in its capacity to promote the balancing of the masculine and feminine energies. The best sex comes when both partners are able to take turns embodying the masculine and feminine elements of sexual union. This allows you to switch roles and practice holding space for both energies through your lovemaking in a safe and open environment.

The partner embodying feminine energy will be relaxed, receptive, and open to being acted upon. Regardless of gender, either partner can play this role while the other is embodying the masculine role of acting. When you are in your feminine energy, you'll be receiving the attentions of your partner as they massage, caress, kiss, and please you. Nurturing your partner during lovemaking is another way to embody the feminine. If you communicate verbally during sex, listening to what is being said and being open to meeting the needs of your partner is a very healing way to embody the feminine.

When embodying the masculine, you will be assertive and active. You will be the one giving foreplay while your partner relaxes and receives your affections. Any time you speak up to assert your needs, whether you want to try something different or communicate to your partner that something is making you uncomfortable, you embody your masculine energy. If you take the dominant role in sex, for instance, taking the top position and moving your body to please your partner while they receive, this can be a very empowering embodiment of the masculine.

Understanding the masculine and feminine energies will allow you and your partner to take turns embodying them. When you consciously switch roles, you will see that it is safe to embrace both aspects of yourself and begin to heal and restore balance. This conscious switching will require you to slow down and allow both partners to act out different roles, which will extend your lovemaking and enhance your libido.

There is a world of pleasure available to those who are willing to be open to trying something new. By consciously working to balance your masculine and feminine energies through lovemaking, you will experience sex as you never have before.

Chapter 7 Spicy And Dirty Talk

She's eating a banana, but as she does, she peels back the skin and takes the banana into her mouth as if it's your dick. What she's trying to say is that eating a banana isn't what's on her mind. The language of dirty talk extends to body language. As her tongue goes over the top of that banana, she isn't thinking of fruit.

When he is rock hard and puts his hand upon your knee, he isn't after a cuddle. Sometimes you have to gage the ferocity of the language. If he's rock hard and ready, don't be a prude. Let him have what he wants and let him have it now. Drop your panties, sit on his lap and whisper dirty words into his ear.

The suggestive things that people do often get unnoticed. She dresses up especially for him but he's still got his mind on work. He brings her flowers but she's too busy on the phone talking to her friend. You need to re-introduce courtesies with your dirty talk. If you know you're in the mood, switch off the phones. If you know you want to catch him by surprise, make sure he's susceptible to it and relaxed. Often people misread the signals. She wants hot sex. He wants to recover from a day's work first. Let him unwind and use subtle dirty talk to see where that leads you. You may be surprised that the slowing down of the whole process actually puts all the obstacles out of the way and neither one of you has to be frustrated by the actions of the other – if forethought is put into the picture.

Walk past him while he's watching TV. Ask if he wants to fondle your breasts. If it's a man that is thinking in sexual terms, the best turn on for a woman knows that he thinks she's the hottest woman around. Drop a chocolate kiss onto her lips and then explore her body. "I can't wait babe, I need you right this moment, here and now." Hold her – let her know that she's the sexiest woman you know. If she says she hasn't got time or needs to be somewhere else, opt for a quickie because these can be every bit as much fun. Up close and dirty, move her to the edge of a table and reach up to take off her panties. "You want a quickie to keep you going until later?" may just get the reaction that you want. You know your woman. You have to be able to know what her response is likely to be. Hot, quick sex can really hit the spot sometimes while at other times passion, foreplay and afterplay are so important.

Dirty talk adds suggestion. It also adds an element of excitement to your love life. "Get into that bedroom wench!" can make her wet on the spot if she is that way inclined. Grabbing him by the tie and leading him to the bed and telling him that you want what you want and are not giving in until you get it can get great results. You don't have to use the "F" word if that makes you uncomfortable, but you can still dirty talk in a subtle way that you both understand is meant to enhance your love lives rather than make them feel tacky and dirty.

Encourage your lover by telling him/her "Oh my, I love it when you do that with your tongue" because otherwise how will your partner ever know. "Do that again but a little to the left" helps him to find the place that really makes you go wild. "Show me what you're made of" is a taunt that will probably result in hard and horny sex. "I want to feel you deep inside me" will probably have similar results.

The problem is that often we are too busy making love to actually comment upon what's being done to us and that's a real shame. How does your partner know what you like? How does he know what you really don't like and what makes you cringe? Praise all those great moments because when you do, you let him know what pleasures you and since your pleasure is his main aim, he will do it more often because you voiced your opinion. That's vital to dirty talk.

Understand how all the different positions affect the depth of sex. If you don't want sex in the standard missionary position, tell him "I'm no missionary – move over mister" and roll on top of him for a change instead of letting sex become tedious. There are two people on the bed and the opinions of both count. "Hey that's so deep," tells him how effective his lovemaking is. Of course, he wants to hear that you feel he's large enough to pleasure you, so there's no harm in subtle dirty talk at all. It boosts his ego and it gets what you want more often.

A guy likes to have his ego stroked, but only if you are genuine. Try to avoid the obvious disaster words – words that are not specific to him or to her. A man who calls all women "darling" doesn't endear himself to his woman. It's not special enough because he uses it all the time and it's not specific enough to her. He could be talking to the girl at the local gas station. Think of horny names that are specific only to you. Similarly, when a girl cries out anything but his name, he's likely to feel a little irked by it. Some people even have randy bedtime names for each other that are hot and affectionate.

The reason I added this chapter was for those who are not accustomed to dirty talk and who are a little nervous about it. The introduction of dirty talk should start with you letting your partner know when something is so right it's pushing all the right buttons. You are complimenting your partner and how crude you want to be depends upon the way that the two of you are accustomed to talking to each other. Dirty talk doesn't have to be demeaning.

"I can feel your sperm squirting inside me"

"Make me cum with your hand!"

"Lick my clitoris until I am all hot and wet and ready for you."

These are words of encouragement. These are words that tell your lover what they are doing right and if you start with encouragement, you may find that you fall into talking dirty with each other simply because it leads on from what you are doing now – which is describing what you want to feel or what he makes you feel inside.

"Play dirty with me, make me cum" isn't something that you should be ashamed of. If he's started to turn you on and he knows that what he is doing is giving you such a lot of pleasure, he will be pleased to oblige. What women need to understand is that men need to be needed. They need to be adored in bed and they also need to acknowledge what they're doing. Otherwise, they may just as well be making love with a blow-up doll. When you both got together, you may have experienced other lovers, but that's not what it's about. Each lover that you have is a totally different, unique human being. By telling your partner what you feel, what you like and what he/she does to pleasure you,

you open up avenues between you to develop that kind of lovemaking so that it's perfect.

It's actually quite endearing to know that the woman is the vamp in bed. That's something that she's good at, but remembers not to call her a "bitch" outside the bedroom because it's bad taste. You need to know the subtleties of the language of love and keep your dirty talk for when it's appropriate. Similarly, he isn't going to respond well at his mother's dining table if you reach your foot up to touch his penis. There are certain times when things are appropriate and times when they are not.

Knowing your partner well enough to know when it's appropriate to use dirty talk is important. There are times when it doesn't work because other things have the priority. Sometimes you both need the language of love and warmth, rather than the pleasure of hot sex with dirty talk, but if you vary your love making, you actually get the best of both worlds.

There's a lot to learn about what dirty talk is all about. Try it and don't knock it until you have. Your man may be very protective toward you, but he may also feel that sometimes it's nice that you take over and let him know what it is that pleasures you.

What women need to remember is that men and women out of bed have different approaches toward life. In bed, basically they want the same thing. Women hold back because they think they should. Men are gentle because they are protective toward their women, but when push comes to shove, a little variation in the bedroom can make the world of difference. If he wants you to be his "whore" in bed, then be it. Be brazen. Be brave and do things that have always been in your mind but you never actually had the guts to do. If she wants you to be masterful, take over. Tie her down to the bed and make her body writhe with pleasure. The language of dirty talk starts when you actually know that your partner accepts you for who you are – rather than who you have been behaving as because of society expectations. No one sees you in bed except him/her. It's a place where inhibitions can be dropped and you can experiment with all kinds of approaches.

If you want to eat strawberry yogurt from the end of his manhood, tell him. Give it your best shot and save a little so that he can have a similar experience in places you want him to explore. The language of love is one that two people can share and if they want to use dirty talk to help them get over the barriers that come between people then it's being used for a very constructive purpose.

Try a word game

Try to think up words that are juicy and sexy and have a contest with him to think of words to describe what it feels like when you cum. Try to think of words that make you horny or words that make you wet. Tell him. There's no shame in it and if you treat it as a game, then it's the prelude to something else. You have created a language of your own that you can pick up on at any time in the future and use to get your wicked way.

People talk about communication being one of the most vital things within a relationship and then get all prudish when it comes to suggesting dirty talk but all dirty talk becomes is an extension to other communication, but you communicate your sexual needs, wants and desires. What other thing can you think of that you can share with your partner that's more intimate, more special?

By exploring the world of dirty talk, you also explore something much deeper than that. You explore your sexuality. You teach your partner what pleases you and learn what pleases your partner. When you have great sex, you begin to realize that it doesn't have to be the same position – the same lead up to sex or the same rolling over and going to sleep after sex. Sex is much more than that. Teach your partner what you like, what you want and what you would actually enjoy and you open up a whole new dialog that helps your communication skills long after you have got out of bed. It's a dynamic to the relationship that is exclusively yours and that's extremely precious. "Make me wet. I want to feel all of you inside me in the shower" could be the start to a new day, and a whole new level of understanding.

Chapter 8 Masturbation

When the fantasy is allowed to flow naturally to the warmth of the hands through the body in search of sensations that lead to satisfying the desire, it is understood why no woman should give up masturbating; Not only for what it means of self-knowledge, but also because it greatly stimulates and deepens enjoyment. In that sense, renowned professionals in the field of medicine and psychology recommend autoeroticism as one of the most authentic and mature forms of sexuality.

Autoerotism awakens at a very early age and manifests itself in adolescence as an intense voluptuous tendency, leading to experiment with the body itself until knowing the hidden springs of sensuality that it ignites.

If self-stimulation is reduced to a simple sexual discharge alone, sexuality is impoverished, since masturbating is always pleasant. And it is not only a substitute for the lover, but it is also an intimate experience that relaxes tensions, avoids stress and contributes to personal serenity and balance. He also teaches and sensually prepares to guide the lover along the path of pleasure through his own body, complementing the erotic games between the two.

How to Enjoy it to the Maximum

A disturbing tickle that runs through the skin in sensual concentric waves that are not located in any area of the body, in particular, indicates to her the presence of desire. It could have caused a presence or a memory, the casual touch of soft underwear or a sentimental song, but whatever the reason, the fantasy begins to fly and gives way to the desire to find an intimate space to self-satisfy.

From that moment, the hands fly entangling themselves in the pubic hair, touching the nipples, crossing the tender line that divides the buttocks in two to reach the pink ring of the anus, and each rub is even more exciting and wakes up a thousand sensations at the same time. From the center of the body rises a heat that at times gains in intensity, the pores of the skin open releasing a thin layer of moisture and a liquid that lubricates it begins to flow, helping to slide the caresses.

The tension in the whole body increases. Little by little, the anxiety grows and, as it happens in all sexual practice, there is not just one unique technique to self-stimulate, but many. Each woman discovers that for herself and that is alternating or changing as you know better.

It is very pleasant to masturbate sitting just on the edge of a surface with your legs open, which allows you to caress the clitoris with one hand and with the other touch the breasts. The perception that intensifies by contracting the PC muscle and leaving the throbbing clitoris, traverses the entire vulva, and notice the sensations that occur in the vagina.

In Solitude

Her imagination is the maximum incentive to stimulate her libido, which makes masturbation one of the most exciting sensual experiences. Nothing prevents her from fantasizing that whoever is working her body has the most ardent and electrifying hands. Visualize your most ardent dreams while stroking, unleashes your excitement. Speak, groan, or scream with pleasure and you can even manage to realize that hidden or forbidden desire in your mind such as a sexual experience with more than one man or with a stranger, or to be taken with violence. You can also imagine risky places where to enjoy sex with the danger of being surprised and a thousand other things. She commands and decides on sexuality alone, is her own guide, her object of desire, and her source of self-satisfaction.

Taken by sensuality, she enjoys penis-shaped sex toys - the dildos - introduces them into the vagina while imagining that he hits her pelvis as she likes while rubbing the clitoris gasping with trembling longing. Images full of hedonism follow one another when a vibrator stimulates the anus or the vagina until it reaches the tense clitoris and its body moves sinuously with intense voluptuousness. Thus stimulated, she soon reaches the threshold of pleasure with her eyes wide open or her eyelids closed firmly rapid breathing, and her heart beating in a hurry until she reaches the pleasant orgasm.

In Couple

Masturbation between lovers is not only one of the games before penetration, but one of the most intense pleasure and probably the one that best contributes to self-knowledge. Nothing prevents her from fantasizing that whoever is going through her body and electrifying her are the hands of the man who excites her. She commands and decides on sexuality alone, is her own guide, her object of desire, and her source of self-satisfaction.

One of the many pleasurable positions to masturbate is to stand in front of a mirror or a fresh wall of tiles and scrub the burning body against it while stimulating the clitoris with one hand and the breasts with the other. Her hand crawls under her clothes looking for the pubis that opens the door to the center of pleasure.

When she is very excited, she begins to wish him to approach the key erogenous points and hint at it in a thousand ways or verbalize it directly, even while she is still dressed. His hand crawls under her clothes looking for the pubis that opens the door to the center of the enjoyment that they both crave. Between the wet hair of desire, he traverses the folds of the vulva with a finger, traces a tense and hot journey through the labia majora, and finally, finds the clitoris that beats anxiously waiting for contact. Her body moves to indicate what excites her most, wishing that the caress rotates, turns, rises, and descends looking for other high centers, while the tongue licks the breasts that she offers yearning.

When he continues to masturbate, she contracts the PC muscle and feels an intense pleasure that extends through the vagina until it climaxes, and if at that point he penetrates her, her orgasm will multiply and become several which will be transported in sensual waves through the whole body, satisfying their desire.

Chapter 9 Orgasms

The word orgasm comes from the Greek word *orgasmos*, which means excitement and swelling. An orgasm in the sudden discharge of accumulated sexual excitement during a sexual session. This discharge results in the rhythmic muscular contraction of the pelvic region and is often described as the height of sexual pleasure in that session.

Orgasm can occur during sex with a partner or during masturbation, and it involves the release of tension in the body. This combination of feeling often goes by many names such as climaxing, cumming, and coming. Orgasming is often characterized by involuntary actions such as muscle spasms, vocalizations, and a general feeling of euphoria.

There are different types of orgasms that a person can experience they include:

- *Tension orgasms.* This results from direct stimulation or results in the release of tension from the body and muscles when it occurs.

- *Multiple orgasms.* This occurs when a series of orgasms occur over a short period of time.

- *Blended orgasms.* This is also called a combination orgasms and results when different types of orgasms are experienced at the same time such as orgasms from oral stimulation and penetration.

- *G-spot orgasms.* These occur from penetrative intercourse and direct stimulation of the erotic zone.

- *Pressure orgasms.* These kinds of orgasms occur from indirect stimulation of applied pressure such as touching through clothing.

- *Relaxation orgasms.* These occur when a body is deeply relaxed during sexual stimulation.

- *Fantasy orgasms.* These result from mental stimulation alone.

There are many biological or physical responses that you will notice when a person orgasms. These responses include:

- Warmth and redness spread across the face and chest.
- Increased breathing rate.
- A quickly beating heart.
- Muscle spasms of the genital and lower abdomen.
- Tension in the thigh and back.
- A rise in blood pressure.
- Temporary loss of motor control.

An orgasm is not just a physical response; it also induces emotional and cognitive changes in the body. Emotional and psychological reactions include:

- Altered states of consciousness.
- Altered states of space and time.
- Activation of the reward pathways in the brain.

- Decrease and inactivation in mental regions associated with behavioral control, anxiety, and fear.

- Feelings of relaxation and happiness.

While these signs and symptoms are general for both males and females, both males and females have decidedly different biological responses to orgasms. Before we get to the characteristics of both male and female orgasms, let's take a moment to look at a few facts concerning orgasms:

- Orgasms have many great benefits apart from the release of sexual tension such as the reduced risk of prostate cancer, pain relief, and even an increased lifespan.

- Orgasms do not only occur during sexual stimulation and can result from everyday activities.

- Orgasms can occur with or without the presence of a condom, and the barrier does not hinder the occurrence of orgasms.

- Women find it harder to reach orgasm compared to men. Up to 40% of women report having difficulty or inability to reach orgasm during sexual stimulation.

- One of the best ways to stimulate a female to orgasm is through clitoral stimulation.
- The quality and frequency of orgasms can improve as women age.
- Self-esteem is a huge factor that influences the occurrence of orgasms during sexual intercourse.
- Women usually take more than 20 minutes to orgasm while it takes a shorter period of time for most men.

Male Orgasms

A male orgasm is only possible after a man gets erect as a result of excitement. Erection occurs when blood flows to the penis causing it to swell in size and become rigid. The testes also become drawn toward the male body. As a result of stimulation, a man's blood pressure will rise, his pulse will quicken, and his rate of breathing increases, all of which are symptoms that he is being sent closer to the ultimate fulfillment.

The act of a man orgasming is called a resolution. It is often thought that males have to ejaculate semen during an orgasm, but it is possible to have an orgasm without ejaculation. When a man does ejaculate during orgasm, he can squirt up to 2 teaspoons of semen, which is a white fluid that contains sperm and other entities.

After a man orgasms, there comes a temporary recovery phase where more orgasms are not possible. This is called a refractory period, and its length varies from man to man, ranging from a few minutes to a few days. Generally, this period becomes longer as a man grows older.

Female Orgasms

Excitement incites the possibility of a woman orgasming. When a woman is sexually excited, blood vessels within her genitals dilate to increase blood flow supply to that region. Her vulva becomes swollen and fluids are secreted from her vaginal canal making her "wet." Just like with a man, her heart rate picks up, high blood pressure rises, and her breathing quickens.

As a woman's excitement begins to plateau, her breasts will increase in size by as much as 25%, and her nipples will become erect. When an orgasm does occur, her genital muscles will experience rhythmic contractions that are less than one second apart. The female orgasm usually averages in length of about 13 to 50 seconds. Ejaculation is not a common symptom when a female orgasms, although it is possible and is sometimes called female ejaculation. It involves the squirting of a clear liquid that is commonly confused with urination, but it is not, and it is not something that a female should be ashamed of or embarrassed to share with her partner.

Women, unlike men, do not experience a refractory period and can have further orgasms if stimulated again.

Different People Orgasm Differently

No matter the symptoms or characteristics that you exhibit during orgasm, there is no right way or wrong way to reach that culmination of feeling. Some people can reach orgasm quickly and easily, while others need more time and stimulation to get to that point. Some positions work best for some, while others can orgasm strictly from penetration. Some people need masturbation or the aid of toys or visual stimulation. All of this and others are perfectly normal and perfectly fine. Go with what feels good to your body, and experiment to find the other ways that make you climax. A good, supportive relationship partner will encourage you to explore your body and its responses to different stimuli and put in the work necessary to bring you pleasure. In response, you should do the same.

As a final note, having an orgasm should not be the ultimate thought when it comes to having sex as it puts too much pressure on reaching that moment. This can make you and your partner anxious. This makes the act of sex stressful and definitely unfulfilling, especially if that ultimate goal is not reached. Relax and let the natural flow of things happen so that you and your partner get the most pleasurable response from sexual intimacy.

Sexual Positions to Incite Male Orgasm

While it is true that men find it easier to orgasm compared to women, there are sex positions that are guaranteed to completely blow his mind. These usually focus on stimulating nerve endings at the tip of his shaft and allow him to build up toward prolonged pleasure.

Prolonged Hand Job

In this instance, it is about making it completely about the man's pleasure. Have him lie down or sit in a reclined position that is comfortable for him while naked. Get between his knees and with a hand and fingers that have been well-lubricated start to stroke his engorged member. Start off by stroking slowly and slowly building strength and speed. Move your hands in an up-and-down motion. You can vary the length and strength of your motions while using one hand or both hands at the same time. If you are using both hands, twist your hands in opposing directions as you move up and down. If the man is circumcised, you can slide the skin of his shaft up and down for added sensation. If he is uncircumcised, move the foreskin back gently and tease the sensitive area just below the tip of his shaft.

Keep eye contact with him as you do this. To make this interlude as pleasurable as possible for the man, pull back or slow the strokes of your hand as you feel his body moving closer to orgasm so that you prolong the drive. This makes the strength of the orgasm stronger when it does finally come.

Do not be afraid to ask him if he likes what you are doing or to show you how exactly he wants the motions of your hand or hands to proceed.

The Sensual Panther

In this position, the woman lies on top and parallel to the man. Her chest and legs are pressed against him. The woman has the leeway of being able to stimulate him in different ways such as kissing along his neck and whispering dirty talk to him. Since her legs are not spread, the penetration in this position is shallow but tight and allows the man to last longer and build up slowly toward a powerful climax.

Turntable

In this position, the woman lies on her side with her legs brought to a 90-degree angle to her upper body. The man lies on top of her just as he would in the missionary position, but the angle of penetration is different since she is lying on her side and he is not between her thighs. This position is great for men because it promotes tightness and pressure around the penis. If the man's penis is curved to the left or right, there is the added bonus that it will stimulate the front or back of the woman's vagina.

Side by Side

This is a position that promotes shallow penetration and, therefore, is great for allowing a man to prolong his climax. In addition, it allows the partners to have lots of eye and skin contact, and so it promotes deeper emotional connections. To get into position, the partners need to lie facing each other. The man's pelvis needs to be slightly lower than the woman's. She will lift her top leg and wrap it around his waist. This position can be thought of as a back to front spoon. The woman may need to tilt her lower body away from the man's or lift her leg higher to allow penetration.

The Cross

In this position, the man lies on his side while the woman slides into a position perpendicular to his body. Her legs will be draped over his hips with her feet ending up behind his buttocks. She needs to press her pelvis against his and open her legs slightly to allow penetration. The man can aid thrusting by gripping the woman's hips and pulling her back and forth on him. He can also reach down to stimulate his partner's clit. This position helps the man last longer because his range of motion is limited and the penetration is shallow.

Modified Sitting in a Chair

In this position, the man sits in a chair and the woman sits on top of him with her back to his front. The woman gets more control in this sex position and can move up and down, grind her pelvis against the man and even use her PC muscles to squeeze his member to her leisure. This position works to prolong the man's pleasure because since the woman is in control, he cannot get carried away. He also has his hands free to touch other parts of her body.

Sexual Positions to Incite Female Orgasm

Women find it harder to orgasm from penetrative sex, but with foreplay and the right position, anything is possible. The sex positions that will be described below promote having the penis stroke the walls of the vagina as well as clitoral stimulation so that the woman has a greater change of climaxing.

Altered X Marks the Spot

This position is wonderful for women since it allows the man's penis to stimulate her G-spot when he penetrates her. This stimulation is facilitated by the upward pressure on her vaginal walls by the tip of the man's penis. To get into position, the woman lies on her back with her knees crossed and her knees brought up to her chest. Her pelvis is braced against the man's thighs and he is able to thrust into her. This position is great for the man, too, since the position requires her to have her thighs closed, which increases the tightness of penetration.

Linguini

To get into this position, the woman lies on her front with her body slightly tilted to one side with one leg slightly raised. The man gets behind her and puts one leg under her raised up so that their lower halves are scissored. This position is great for women since it not only allows the man to stimulate her G-spot with his thrusts but she can also have her clitoris stimulated by grinding against the man's thigh. The man benefits, as well, since the position promotes greater tightness around his penis.

Standing Delivery

In this position, both parties are standing. The woman is in front and faces away from the man. To align their pelvises, one party may need to bend their knees depending on who is taller. Once the pelvises are aligned, penetration can be achieved. This position is great for promoting female orgasm since the clitoris is easily accessed. The man can also play with other parts of the woman like her breasts and other erogenous zones in her front while being able to kiss her neck and lips if she tilts her head toward him. The man also can have an amazing orgasm since there is increased friction and tightness due to the angle of penetration.

Sitting Scissors

In this position, the man sits and the woman gets on top. She kneels with her back to his front and places one leg on the outside of the man's body and the other leg between the man's legs. She then fits her pelvis against the man's to allow penetration. Women find it easier to orgasm in this position because they can control the length and depth of penetration in addition to having their clit stimulated by themselves or by the man. The man can also increase the pleasurable sensations the woman feels by playing with breasts and kissing her neck and back. The man can also lie back to vary the depth and angle of penetration.

Sideways Straddle

This is a girl on top position. The woman kneels facing away from the man with her knees on either side on one of his legs. The man needs to raise this leg so that it presses against the woman's clitoris. The woman can use her hands to guide the man's penis into her vagina. Women love this position for the obvious clitoral stimulation as well as being able to control the intensity and depth of penetration.

Chapter 10 Sex Toys: What Choose For Him And For Her

The first sex toy I ever used was a dildo. After that, a trip to the sex shop for Valentine's Day started a couple month long foray into the incorporation of toys into my sex life. It's one of the best decisions I ever made.

They are not only a quick and efficient way to take your sex life to the next level, but they're super fun to mess around with. They can do things we simply can't do, or at least not as skillfully (like vibrate).

However, it's important not to think of them as REPLACEMENTS, but rather ENHANCEMENTS of you, your partner(s), and the sex life you already have together.

The name of the game is pleasure, connection, fun, and intimacy. Sex toys help with all of that. By themselves, they can only accomplish a mere fraction of it.

So for people who are hesitant to venture into the world of these devices because of an insecurity you have about them (like I had), trust me when I say it's completely unfounded and you are truly missing out on an exciting aspect of sexuality, not to mention you may be leaving your partner hanging.

There are a number of directions I could have gone with this chapter, but I decided to focus it purely on using sex toys while having sex itself. I also decided to focus on how to use them to optimize the pleasure of both partners.

There are TONS to choose from. It can be quite daunting the moment you step into the sex shop or the online store loads on your computer screen.

Dildos, vibrators, BDSM devices, masturbators, anal stimulators, dolls, edible underpants – the list goes on and on. And within each type of toy are different sub-categories meant for different pleasure goals. So how am I going to narrow this down?

I'm only going to go over the main ones. Why? Because once you understand how they work and have experienced them, that's when you gain a strong enough background knowledge to choose the ones that are REALLY going to enhance your experience.

You will also feel much more comfortable starting out with these than some of the more intricate ones. I've also included links to examples of each to give you a better idea of what I'm talking about.

Diddling Around with Dildos

Dildos are typically made out of a silicone, silicone-type material, or glass and have a phallic shape (the general shape of a penis).

It's a good beginner's toy because it's not complicated to figure out how to use it. If you have a penis, you already know how. Use it like you would your penis.

The following suggestions can be practiced as a part of foreplay, as a break from intercourse in the middle of a session, or whenever it tickles your fancy.

- If you're using a dildo on your partner and they haven't been penetrated yet, enter them slowly and be attentive to how they react. Using a good amount of lube is also recommended.

- Angle the toy towards the G-Spot and/or prostate for maximum pleasure. It can also be used to stimulate the clitoris and/or outer part of the anus or perineum as well.

- In the case of penetrative sex for those who have a vagina, dildos can be used for double penetration (stimulating the vagina with the penis, and the anus with the dildo) or the other way around.

- Strap-on dildos also fall under this category and can be used in any of the above ways.

- You can also find double-penetration dildos, which can be used to stimulate one partner or to be shared between two partners (be aware of hygiene concerns).

- Dildos can also have a vibrating component. The most common are "rabbit" vibrating dildos which have a protrusion from one side, meant to stimulate either the clitoris or the anus.

- There are also dildos meant for anal stimulation. The most common are referred to as "butt plugs," and have a splayed bottom so the toy doesn't get lodged inside the rectum.

Example dildos to check out:

- *Glass Dildo with Ribbed Sides*
- *"Rabbit" Dildo with Vibration*

Vibrators – Bite-sized Pleasure That Packs a Punch

Vibrators are usually made of plastic and generally come in smaller sizes. But these little Energizer Bunny sex toys pack a powerful punch.

For many, and those who have vaginas especially, the use of a vibrator is one of the only ways they can orgasm during intercourse. For some, this includes masturbation as well.

Either way, using vibrators is one of the best ways to enhance your sex.

- A torpedo vibrator comes in the shape of a miniature torpedo. They're about 2-4 inches in length and are one of the most common vibrators.

- Typically, vibrators have different settings that allow you to adjust the speed and intensity of the vibration.

- For those who have a vagina, focus most of your efforts on and around the clitoris. Pay attention to how your partner is reacting. When using a vibrator, the clitoris can become overstimulated rather quickly. Stimulation above, to the side, and on the sensitive tissue below the clitoris might be more pleasurable for your partner.

- For those with a penis, using a vibrator on the head and/or testicles can be pleasurable as well.

- For anal play, focus vibration where the highest density of nerve endings are – the outer tissue, inner two-thirds, and the prostate or area close to the G-Spot.

- Vibrators truly stand out during sexual intercourse. As long as you are in a position where either you or your partner can reach a hand to a part of the other partner's genitals, vibrators can be used. For G-Spot or prostate stimulation, I have found that the best position is either missionary or the first position we described, "Missionary With Legs in the Air." During these positions, penetration is providing intense stimulation on the inner part of the genitals, so you can intensify the experience by using a vibrator to stimulate the outer part of the genitals.

Example vibrators to check out:

- *Typical Torpedo Vibrator*
- *A Popular Type of Massage Vibrator*
- *Dual-Stimulation Vibrator*

Vibrating Rings

Commonly called "penis rings," vibrating rings are just as their name describes – rings that vibrate. Don't worry, they're elastic and usually the part that vibrates is protruding outward.

- For penetrative sex, wearing the ring over the object that is penetrating can add pleasure for both partners.

- For the receiving partner, make sure the ring is positioned so it can make contact with your genitals as your partner thrusts. It should also make the entire penetrating object vibrate as well.

- As the penetrating partner, it's your job to control the stimulation. Rather than constant continuous thrusting, try slow and careful movements. Pause when you are all the way in and the ring has made contact with your partner. Allow the feeling to soak in. Then pull out suddenly, and move in extremely slowly again, teasing your partner. They'll be dying for you to go all the way in. Make them crave it before giving it to them. Don't forget our old motto of give and take.

- You can also find tongue vibrating rings which are meant for cunnilingus. In my experience, they flat out suck, so I wouldn't spend too much money if you plan on buying one. It's an awesome concept, but the execution is awful. Using it is almost like performing cunnilingus while your tongue is numb, because you can't feel what you're touching. I wouldn't recommend it, but hey, maybe you will be more skilled than me.

Example vibrating rings to check out:

- *Trojan Brand Vibrating Ring*
- *Classic Vibrating Ring*
- *Vibrating Tongue Ring*

Kinky and Restrictive Devices

Constraint is a turn on for many people. It helps define and play out the sexual roles of domination and submission. However, a common complaint is one partner wanting to kink up their sex life while the other doesn't feel comfortable with it.

There are numerous psychological reasons behind this. But the bottom line is that you two should progress slowly, carefully, and supportively. Both partners need to have a high level of trust and must know when to stop before things go too far.

That being said, there are some fun introductory items to use that aren't too crazy and will still add an entirely new dynamic to your sex life.

- **Blindfolds**. Putting a blindfold on one partner can be extremely sexy. The partner that's blindfolded is suddenly engorged in a world of mystery, while the other is given the perfect opportunity to be creative. Their partner won't know what's about to happen to them until it happens. The partner without the blindfold should take this opportunity to tease them like crazy. Run your fingers up their body. Barely graze over their private parts. Make them crave knowing what's going to happen next. Then make it happen. Again, the level of trust must be high, but this is a great place to start.
- **Rope Ties**. As far as constraint goes, rope ties should be your first stop. You can tie up any appendages and restrict their range of motion. By doing this, you give your partner something to flex

against while they're being stimulated, which can help them orgasm. There is also a lot of cognitive pleasure involved, as one partner submits control to the other. It's a fun way to play out certain fantasies. However, proceed with caution. Tying people up certain ways can cause injury.

- **Handcuffs.** These provide similar pleasure to rope ties, but the cognitive pleasure of being handcuffed is different from being tied up. Handcuffs are usually made of metal as well, which can be painful. Try to find a pair that has a cushiony or protective covering.

Example kinky and restrictive devices to check out:

- *Padded Leather Blindfold*
- *Rope Tie and Vibrating Dildo*
- *Cushioned Handcuffs*

Those are the main introductory toys that I decided to include. Of course, there are loads more. A quick Google search is evidence of that.

If you would like to check out more of what's out there, here are a few online stores:

- *Adam and Eve*
- <u>*Spencer's*</u>
- *Pure Romance*
- *Amazon – Sex Toys Department*

Look at sex toys as a way to introduce a kinkier side to your sex life. Challenge yourself to see just how high you can increase the pleasure of you and your partner. It's an interesting endeavor, and worthwhile once you take the plunge.

This next chapter discusses something that literally changed my sex life in one night.

Enough said.

Chapter 11 Using Props During Sex

The ideas in this chapter are just suggestions to start with. Feel free to experiment with your partner and find out what excites you both!

Props to Set the Mood

One very easy way to use props during sex is to use them to set the mood. A bedroom that is sensually decorated is a perfect reminder to you and your partner to save a little time for yourselves, and you can also use special decorations for times when you want to surprise your partner or have a particularly memorable evening. There are many different ways to use props to create the sexual atmosphere that you and your partner desire. Candles, in particular, are a nice way to turn an ordinary bedroom into a sexy boudoir. Scented candles can make the room smell wonderful, while the low lighting invites sexual advances. For those with a sense of humor, there are also fun, phallic candles that can be found online or at your local sex shop. Decorate to set the mood that you want to create!

Vibrators and Dildos

Many people may think that vibrators and dildos are for masturbation and not useful while having sex with a partner, but these toys can actually be a fun addition to a couple's sex life. Vibrators can be added in as a couple has penetrative sex, particularly in positions where the woman is able to stimulate her own clitoris. Many women have trouble achieving an orgasm with penetrative vaginal stimulation alone, so using a vibrator while having sex can help to ensure that she has just as much fun as he does. He can also use a vibrator on her as they have sex. Try using a vibrator during some of the positions in chapters 1, 2, and 3 of this book, such as Ride 'Em, Ladies and Puppy Love (Easy), All About Legs, Take a Ride in Reverse, and Keeping it Erect (Intermediate), and Come From Behind (Advanced).

Vibrators and dildos can also be a great addition to mutual masturbation. Some men find it difficult to provide intense enough stimulation to the clitoris with their fingers to bring a woman to orgasm. A vibrator can help in these situations. In addition, some women like the feeling of their vaginal opening being stretched very wide, even wider than most men's penises can physically get. Men shouldn't be offended by this, but rather treat it as an opportunity to use a dildo and get the woman very turned on before having penetrative sex. Some women like the feel of a dildo when it is inserted and does not move, while others like an in-and-out movement more similar to sex. Communication is key for unlocking the possibilities of vibrators and dildos!

Using Food as a Prop

Food is one of the best classic erotic props due to its availability and the endless possibilities that come with incorporating it into sex. It might be a little daunting to walk into a sex shop and purchase a vibrator, but it's not in the least difficult to go to your local grocery store and buy some whipping cream. If you and your partner are looking to mix up your sex life without getting too daring, using food as a prop is a perfect place to start.

One of the easiest ways to use food as a prop is to incorporate it into erotic massage and foreplay. Try covering your partner's body or sensitive areas with a creamy or spreadable food and then licking them all over until they are clean. You can use whatever food you prefer, but some easily used foods are whipping cream, chocolate syrup, marshmallow creme, peanut or almond butter, chocolate hazelnut spread, jams or jellies, and frosting. You might want to put down a towel beforehand or plan to change the sheets afterward!

Ice is one of the most flexible foods when it comes to sex. To avoid the uncomfortable sticking sensation of very cold ice on the skin, use "warm ice," which has been out of the freezer 10-20 minutes and is starting to melt. You can run ice cubes up and down your partner's body, concentrating on their erogenous zones. You can also put ice cubes in your mouth and then put your mouth on your partner's body, even during oral sex. This can produce very different and exciting sensations. It's also possible to insert ice cubes into a female partner's vagina. Just make sure to use warm ice when you do this since very cold ice can have sharp edges that can be painful.

Another way to incorporate food into sex is to feed one another. It's highly dubious that any foods (oysters, dark chocolate, ginger, or otherwise) actually affect libido, but some people are turned on by feeding a partner or by getting fed by a partner. The easiest way to try this is to start with easy-t0-eat foods in bite size pieces. Pieces of fruit, small chocolates, or nuts are a good place to start. Eating or feeding your partner too much of a heavy food may make you or them less willing to have sex since they may start to feel unwell, so be careful. Otherwise, find out what you and your partner like, and have fun!

One important consideration when using food as a prop during sex is to not insert any food into the vagina that may get stuck there. People certainly have used particular kinds of vegetables as dildos, but it's a lot safer just to go and buy a sex toy. A dildo made to be inserted into the vagina is unlikely to break off and get stuck there, unlike a carrot, for example. Vegetables are also organic matter and can carry bacteria that is not good for the vagina. The same is true for candies, which have the added problem of being very sugary. This sugar attracts unhealthy bacteria, which can lead to infections. In general, if you and your partner would like to insert an object other than a penis into the vagina, use a dildo, a vibrator, or ice, since it will simply melt into water rather than getting stuck.

Other Sex Toys

There is a huge variety of other sex toys that you and your partner can incorporate into your sex lives. Many of these toys can be found at a sex shop or online. A sex shop may be embarrassing to visit, but rest assured that there is nothing shameful about enjoying sex and using toys. By going to a sex shop, you can get a better idea of what a toy looks like and if it is good quality or not. Going online can be less stressful, but you run the risk of ending up with a poor-quality toy. When it comes to sex toys, it's always better to spend a little extra money to get a quality item. You don't want yourself or your partner to get hurt using a cheap toy.

Many sex toys are bondage-type toys that can heighten the excitement for couples, especially those who enjoy dominant/submissive sex play. Blindfolding your partner, handcuffing them, or tying them to the bedposts are all ways to incorporate this type of toy. You can find special blindfolds, handcuffs, and ropes for use during sex, which is a good idea because everyday versions of these items are not always well-suited for sex play.

Other sex toys are meant to add to the sensation produced by the penis during penetrative sex. The simplest of these toys are specialty condoms, which can usually be purchased at drugstores. These condoms have extra ridges, bumps, or textures, which can be fun for women. More specialized toys include penis extenders, some of which also include extra bumps and ridges, and strap-ons, which allow for a woman to penetrate a man anally. If you and your partner are interested in some of these more elaborate toys, it could be fun and sexy to visit a sex shop together and pick out a toy to use together. You'll both be looking forward to getting home to try it out!

A final consideration for all sex toys: make sure you are cleaning them well and not sharing them with others! Sex toys, especially those that penetrate the body, should be personalized. Sharing these toys could transmit infections, particularly STI's, so be careful, keep your toys clean, and stay safe!

Chapter 12 Sexual And Aphrodisiac Food

Choosing the right food is easy because every religion and every culture have their share of special food. One can choose from common vegetables and fruits like broccoli, artichoke, leafy greens onion, ginger, and eggplant. These help the juices flow. Here you will see some popular food items.

Eat the right foods

For having good sex that is satisfying you need to have a good flow both through your blood vessels and through your sex organs. You need to satisfy your sex fantasies, so eat well. Foods that increase the flow of blood, testosterone and estrogen are available from our grocery shop. Eating these types of fruits and vegetables will keep you in fit condition always. Your sexual intercourse will be vigorous and satisfying. Here are some of these "sexy foods".

Chocolate

Chocolate dates back a long way in history to the times of Casanova and Louise the XV in terms of being used for stimulating the passions. However, this is applicable only to dark chocolate or at the least containing 70% or more of dark chocolate. The magic ingredient in chocolate that helps boost your senses is phenyl ethylamine. Keep a few pieces in the back of the cupboard for those times when you are feeling low.

Horseradish

This food item is quite popular in Japan. People eat it with their sushi and this side dish packs a wallop in the excitation department. Check out the items in your nearest mall, you might get lucky.

Chili Peppers: This spice helps boost the metabolic rate, meaning it gets the blood flowing. This supposedly triggers the release of endorphins that puts you 'in the mood'.

Oysters: Famous since the olden ages as an aphrodisiac, oysters have zinc in them that is beneficial for the production of testosterone. This increases the sex drive in both men and women.

Women get easily "into the mood" when they have oysters.

Nuts: Pine nuts help your libido. They are good for your brain too. Nuts like almonds have plenty of essential amino acids that help to keep sex hormones thriving. Brazil nuts will benefit men more because the selenium content will keep the health of the sperm cells intact.

Caviar: Caviar is fish eggs that have plenty of vitamins. Many people have a sex fantasy that involves caviar. It has phosphorus that makes your nerves steady and active. The best combination for caviar is vodka. But do not drink too much vodka, only a little, or you may have trouble maintaining an erection.

Avocado: Since the time of the Aztecs, avocados have been accepted as one major fruit that increases a person's vitalistic energy. The very shape of the fruit is sensuous and delicious; over the past few years, scientists have been studying how much of an aphrodisiac the fruit actually is. Despite the fact the research is still being conducted, the fact remains that avocado contains high levels of Vitamin E and helps you retain an energy level that is unprecedented.

Honey: The very idea of honey is something that sparks a sensuous image in our heads; not for nothing do we call sex 'the birds and the bees'. It has long since served as a symbol of procreation in literature and art, but the fact is adding a few spoons of honey to your daily diet will boost your sex life unimaginably! It contains the nutrient boron, which not only gives you a natural energy boost but also regulates your estrogen and testosterone levels, so use honey creatively in food as well as your lovemaking!

Pine Nuts

Doctors, having studied these little gems over years, suggest that pine nuts are incredibly helpful in maintaining an active and healthy sex life. This is because they are rich in zinc, which is a highly energizing mineral that leads to a powerful sex drive. Just extracting these nuts from pinecones is hard enough, so be sure to add it to your diet to boost your sex life!

Arugula

This exotic sounding plant is a food that has been documented as an aphrodisiac since early times. It contains a host of minerals and antioxidants; like a number of its other leafy green counterparts, this plant counters the effects of any toxic substances that your body has absorbed from the environment that kills your libido. It boosts your immunity, thereby increasing overall energy levels and vitality.

Olive Oil

Not only is olive oil a much healthier option to cook with, it helps with your sex drive as well! It is rich in antioxidants and is an excellent source of both monounsaturated as well as polyunsaturated fats – these fats keep your blood flow pumping, your heart healthy and aid in the regulation and production of hormones too! The Greeks believed that olive oil makes men that much more virile; whether this is true or not is still under research, but the fact is that it increases overall energy and boost vitality, which is always brilliant for a healthy sex drive!

Pomegranates

Looking sensuous and exotic from the get go, pomegranates are some of the most nutritious fruits around. They are rich in antioxidants and support a powerful blood flow, making sure that you are energized and stay healthy. One study found that eating pomegranates on a regular basis helps men with erectile dysfunction, so go ahead and add it to your diet! Plus, there is nothing quite like eating these seeds off your lover's body.

Pumpkin Seeds

These little gems are rich in magnesium content – in fact, they are perhaps the richest in magnesium in most food categories. Magnesium, when taken in the right dosage, is brilliant for an active sex life – it increases the testosterone levels by making sure that more amount of testosterone enters your blood streams and keeps it flowing.

Drinks Champagne or red wine helps boost the sex drive. But too much alcohol is not recommended as it can affect your sex drive adversely.

Bananas

This fruit contains plenty of phosphorus and chelating minerals. This helps improve libido. In addition, it contains plenty of vitamins. So, if you have nothing else to try out, go for bananas to make your night wild.

Exercise daily

Wake up early in the morning. Use any mechanism possible but rise up and do some meditation. This makes your mind free from negative thoughts. First, the movement of your limbs and body will shake up your internal organs. It will revitalize them and improve the blood flow. You burn up the excess energy that would otherwise become fat. This makes you hungrier and your metabolism improves.

Plan your itinerary

It helps if you keep a watch over your daily schedule. If you set aside ten minutes for a walk, it makes you mentally prepared every day for the walk. In the same way, if you set aside thirty to forty minutes for lovemaking, it will help your mind to get attuned to the activity. After a few days, you can make adjustments to this item by adding time or adding the type of sexual intercourse you will be doing.

Chapter 13 The Intricacies of Pleasure and Orgasms

What is pleasure, in its simplest form?

It's the enjoyable feeling of satisfaction you receive when a desire is fulfilled.

When you've been craving a slice of pizza all day, and you get off work, head straight to Pizza Hut, wait patiently for your order to finish, and take that first cheesy, meaty, greasy, glorious bite, THAT feeling right there is pleasure.

Psychology describes pleasure in terms of positive feedback. We are motivated to seek out what gives us pleasure and recreate those instances that have given us pleasure in the past.

For our purposes, first we need to understand pleasure in its physical form (although, its mental form is just as important, and we will see how the two cooperate).

Physical pleasure stems from our central nervous system, the network of neurons that transmit information from all parts of our bodies to our brains.

Nerve endings near the surface of our skin receive these signals first. The density of these nerve endings differ in various parts of our body.

Can you guess where one of the highest concentrations might be?

If you guessed your genitals, you just won the $1 million prize. Well, maybe just a million orgasms (I'd rather have the latter).

According to Ian Kerner, Ph. D., sex counselor, and best-selling author of She Comes First: The Thinking Man's Guide to Pleasuring a Woman, the penis contains about 4,000 nerve endings while the clitoris contains about 8,000 (he doesn't note how many in the whole vagina/vulva, but there are more in the outer lips, inner lips, vaginal entrance, and inside the vagina).

That's A LOT. It's no wonder these areas are so sensitive.

You may be thinking, "Alright cool, I'll just focus on mine and my partner's genitals the whole time and we will have amazing orgasms. That's what I figured anyway."

It's not that simple, or that boring. Sexual pleasure is complex, but that is what makes it such an exciting journey to navigate.

I prefer to think less in terms of having sex with my partner's body, and more in terms of having sex with their brain and their mind as well.

I know that sounds strange, but it makes sense considering the brain is where all of our pleasure signals end up.

Breaking Down Orgasms

The road to orgasm is navigated in terms of phases, with mental and physical pleasure playing a part throughout.

Sex researchers, Masters and Johnson, identified four stages to what they call the "sexual response cycle." These stages are Excitement, Plateau, Orgasm, and Resolution.

The following derives from WebMD, sprinkled with my take on each phase.

Stage 1 – Excitement (time frame: A few minutes to several hours)

This is when your body and mind recognize that **sexual tension is present.**

There are palpable sexual overtones, like when you are dancing with someone at a club, or holding hands walking home together, or lying in bed kissing and rubbing each other.

At this point, muscle tension increases. Sometimes you are not consciously aware of it, but your stomach may have tightened or your leg muscles may have stiffened up.

Your heart rate increases and your breathing becomes deeper.

WebMD states that your skin may become flushed, as in reddish blotches around the chest and back. (I have read this before, but I have never seen or noticed it. I have felt my skin getting warmer, however.)

The nipples harden (woot woot!).

Here's the big one: Blood flow to the genitals increases. The penis becomes erect and the clitoris/inner lips swell. Vaginal lubrication also begins (the vulva, or outer area of the vagina including the lips, clitoris, and vaginal entrance, gets "wet").

Breasts gain in size and the internal vaginal walls start to swell. Testicles also swell, the scrotum tightens, and fluid may secrete from the penis.

Phew!

Now that we're all excited, let's move on to Stage 2.

Stage 2 — Plateau

The plateau is everything from initial stimulation to the moment just before release, or orgasm.

You can view this whole process as a constant buildup of sexual tension, through teasing, give and take, multitasking, and some of the other techniques we'll discuss later which make up the meat of this guide.

In this phase, all of the changes that started in the Excitement phase increase in intensity.

The vulva swells further as blood flow increases. The clitoris becomes more sensitive, and may retract under the clitoral hood if it is overstimulated.

The testicles withdraw into the scrotum, and the penis reaches its maximum erection.

Your breathing, heart rate, and blood pressure increase. (What's interesting to note is that this happens even if the person isn't doing any physical activity during sex. I find that to be strong biological evidence for this part of the response cycle).

Muscle spasms may start to occur in places like the feet, face, hands, and thighs. Muscle tension increases further as well.

Stage 3 — Orgasm

The Big O. The Grand Finale. The Whole Shebang. The Thing We All Live For.

Ooorrrgaasmm.

It's when all of that built up tension and desire is released in one (and sometimes multiple) wave of intense feeling and pleasure. Hormones and endorphins flood the brain in a way that can only be described as pure ecstasy.

It's. Awesome.

And it's awesome giving it to someone else as well, but we'll get to that later.

What happens when we have an orgasm?

Involuntary muscle contractions begin, sometimes quite violently. Heart rate, blood pressure, and breathing reach their peak of intensity.

Muscles in the vagina contract, and the uterus also begins to contract.

Muscles contract at the base of the penis stimulating the ejaculation of semen.

Neurohormones (oxytocin and prolactin) are released, which are largely attributed to our feelings of intense pleasure when we have an orgasm. Endorphins are also released, contributing to the same result.

A reddish flush may appear all over the body, especially in the face.

Stage 4 — Resolution

Resolution is the comedown after climax. It's when your body's responses return back to their pre-excitement phase – i.e. back to normal.

It's also when you get that "Ahhhhh..." feeling of relaxation. Your muscles feel like jello, they are just tired enough to be fatigued, and you may feel heightened intimacy with your partner.

The *refractory period* also kicks in at this point. This is the period between the most recent orgasm and when the individual is physically capable of having another one or continuing stimulation.

It's a period where the person needs to rest and recuperate before they can continue more sexual activity.

This period differs for everyone, and even on a circumstantial basis and/or with age, but it is commonly an extended period of time for partners who have a penis. Ever heard partners of those who have a penis complain that their partner falls asleep or can't continue after having an orgasm? The refractory period plays a part in this.

It's important to note that everyone goes through these phases differently and feels them to varying degrees. While there may be a general framework for how everyone progresses to orgasm, we all feel physical pleasure differently, just how people gain pleasure from other things differently, such as pizza.

(I personally don't gain any pleasure from mushrooms. Italian sausage on the other hand…..wait a second. I'll be right back).

That's why communication about what each other likes is so important. It's also why different partners require, and offer a chance at, unique ways to bring them to the highest heights of pleasure.

You also feel pleasure differently than any partners your current partner may have had, so don't forget to tell them what works best for you as well.

As you may have noticed, the physical responses described in the sexual response cycle are largely involuntary. But they are just that – responses to the stimulation of an external force, whether you are stimulating yourself or someone else is stimulating you, and vice versa.

While specific pleasure responses are far from universal, there are MANY aspects of sex that can be applied to any situation.

This book is largely based on the techniques people can use to confidently find the right combination of sexual vehicles that will lead to great sex.

Great sex with most, if not any partner.

On to the meat of this guide: The need-to-knows of foreplay, oral sex, anal sex, powerful sex positions, sex toys, and dirty talk.

This portion of the guide is quite detailed. If you start to feel overwhelmed, read through it slowly, note the important points, and refer to it later when your mind has given the information a chance to sink in.

Chapter 14 The Most Intimate Positions For Couple

When you search for sex positions on the internet, you will find that most sources list the same positions over and over again. While this isn't necessarily a bad thing, they typically don't tell you why they chose them.

For our purposes, I'm only going to include the best of the best that I've found. These are the positions that provide the most pleasure, the hottest sex, the deepest intimacy, and give you the best opportunities to multitask (which will be discussed in a later chapter).

I have broken them up into penetrative, non-penetrative, and oral sex positions. Penetrative includes any object, such as a penis, toy, or strap-on dildo, being used to enter your partner. Non-penetrative includes the rubbing together of genitals and mutual masturbation.

I'll be describing the positions in terms of how both partners should be situated and what benefits each position offers.

Good sex requires different positions. Great sex requires POWERFUL positions.

Let's break 'em down.

Powerful Penetrative Positions

#1 Missionary With Legs in the Air

Description-

- The penetrating partner is on top and the receiving partner is on bottom.

- Instead of regular missionary with the receiving partner's legs spread out on the bed, the receiving partner spreads their legs about two feet apart and lifts them up in the air towards the ceiling, keeping them in front of their partner. Their body becomes an L shape.

- The receiving partner rests the back of their legs against the chest and shoulders of their partner, typically with their knees bending over their partner's shoulders and their hamstrings on their partner's chest.

- The penetrating partner leans forward, with their head between their partner's legs, and put their hands on the bed next to their partner's head, with their arms straight. This should angle their partner's pelvis upwards.
- Finally, the penetrating partner enters.

Benefits-

- Great angle for stimulating the G-Spot, anus, and/or prostate.
- The pressure of the receiving partner's legs provides some relief for the penetrating partner's arms.
- The receiving partner is somewhat constrained, which can be a turn on for many people.

Variation-

- Instead of two legs towards the ceiling, the receiving partner only puts one of their legs up, providing a different angle of stimulation.

#2 Missionary While Grabbing the Butt

Description-

- Regular missionary position with the penetrating partner on top and receiving partner on bottom, except the penetrating partner lies completely on top, resting their weight on their partner.

- With their head to the side of their partner's head, possibly resting on the pillow, the penetrating partner reaches down with both hands and grabs hold of their partner's butt.

Benefits-

- Allows the penetrating partner to pull their partner in towards them and thrust at the same time.

- Creates more bodily contact, increasing intimacy.

- Better angle than regular missionary for stimulating the G-Spot, anus, and/or prostate.

#3 Receiving Partner Lying Sideways and Penetrating Partner On Top

Description-

- The receiving partner lies on their side with legs bent at a 90 degree angle.
- The penetrating partner enters from the top, so the front of the penetrating partner is facing the side of the receiving partner.
- The penetrating partner kneels within the 90 degree angle of their partner's legs, positioning their pelvis to enter their partner.
- The penetrating partner leans forward and places their hands, arms, or elbows on both sides of their partner to hold themselves up.

Benefits-

- Different angle of stimulation.
- Can still kiss each other, heightening intimacy.

Variation-

- The penetrating partner grabs their partner's top leg and puts it over the corresponding arm.
- This widens either the vagina or anus for easier entry, and creates a different dynamic of constraint.

#4 Legs in the Air on the Edge of the Bed

Description-

- Similar to #1. The receiving partner lies on their back, puts their legs **together** and raises them up to the ceiling so their body is in an L shape. Except this time, they are on the edge of the bed with the penetrating partner standing up.

- The penetrating partner wraps or holds on to their partner's legs for thrusting leverage, and may have to bend their knees down a bit to enter their partner. However, this partner does not lean over yet, like in #1, but stays standing straight.

Benefits-

- The penetrating partner gets great leverage by holding onto or wrapping around their partner's legs.
- Another optimal angle for stimulating the G-Spot, anus, and/or prostate.

Variation-

- Can have legs spread open rather than together.
- Can do the same as #1, with legs spread, hamstrings against the chest, and

penetrating partner leaning over their partner while holding themselves up.

#5 Doggy Style With Receiving Partner Curling Towards Other Partner

Description-

- Receiving partner goes on their hands and knees while the penetrating partner gets on their knees and enters from behind.
- Instead of being on their hands, the receiving partner then rests one shoulder on the bed and angles their head to the opposite side, angling their back downwards towards the bed. The receiving partner should be able to look back and see their partner.
- The receiving partner rests their arms on the bed towards their partner.
- The penetrating partner holds on to their partner's hips for thrusting leverage.

Benefits-

- Better angle for deeper penetration.
- Increased arousal by both partners being able to lock eyes with one another, and especially for the receiving partner who gets to see their partner entering them from behind.
- Penetrating partner can get good leverage by holding onto their partner's hips and waist.

Variation-

- The receiving partner bends their knees further and lowers their pelvis down closer to the bed. They then reach back with their hands and wrap their arms around their legs, curling themselves further into a ball.

#6 Doggy Style With Penetrating Partner Squatting Over

Description-

- The receiving partner is on their hands and knees in doggy style position.
- Instead of being on their knees as well, the penetrating partner stands with their feet on either side of their partner, squatting down until they are at the right height to enter. The receiving partner may need to angle their pelvis upwards to help with entry.
- If the penetrating partner is comfortable, they can thrust like this. Otherwise, if they need more balance they can place their hands on the back, shoulders, or hips of their partner while squatting.

Benefits-

- Allows for deeper penetration.

- This angle from behind is better for hitting the G-Spot, anus, and/or prostate.
- The penetrating partner can use gravity to help them thrust.

Variation-

- Similar to the previous position (#5 - Doggy Style With Receiving Partner Curling Towards Other Partner), the receiving partner can angle their back down towards the bed, reach their arms back towards their partner, and curl themselves into a ball. This allows for further comfort during deep penetration and a different angle of stimulation. It also increases intimacy by being able to see each other's faces.

#7 From Behind With Receiving Partner Laying On Stomach

Description-

- The receiving partner lies flat on their stomach with their legs out straight and close together.

- The penetrating partner straddles their partner, with their knees on either side, leans forward, and uses their hands and arms to hold them up while entering their partner.

Benefits-

- Makes the vagina/anus tighten for increased pleasure of both partners.

- A comfortable position for both partners.

- Allows for a lot of multitasking, including hair pulling, kissing and sucking the neck/back, and manual stimulation (hand) of the genitals of the receiving partner.

Variation-

- The penetrating partner lies fully on the receiving partner, without holding themselves up, increasing bodily contact and intimacy.
- The penetrating partner can also reach under and provide manual stimulation to their partner's genitals.
- Provides opportunity to kiss from behind.

#8 Lying Down Sideways Penetration From Behind

Description-

- The receiving partner lies on their side with knees bent at around and 90 degree angle.
- The penetrating partner lies on their side behind them, entering as they would in regular doggy style and using their partner's hip(s) as leverage.

Benefits-

- Hugely intimate position, as it resembles cuddling.

- Provides a lot of opportunity for multitasking, including hair pulling, kissing from behind, manual stimulation of the genitals, and constraint by pulling back and locking the receiving partner's arms.

Variation-

- The penetrating partner lifts up the top leg of the receiving partner, either holding it up or placing it on top of their own. This expands the vagina/anus allowing for more comfortable penetration.

#9 Receiving Partner On Top (with variations)

Description-

- The penetrating partner lies on their back with the receiving partner straddling them.
- The receiving partner sits on their partner as they enter them.
- The receiving partner moves their body in a way that stimulates both partners.

Benefits-

- The receiving partner gets to control rhythm and stimulation.
- The receiving partner gains a more dominant role and can exercise more control.
- The penetrating partner becomes the more submissive role.

- The receiving partner is able to move in a way that best stimulates them, and can control the depth of penetration.

- Provides opportunity for either partner to manually stimulate the receiving partner's genitals in addition to penetration.

Variations-

- Instead of straddling their partner on their knees, the receiving partner squats over, bending their knees far enough to have their partner enter them. They can place their hands on their partner's shoulders, chest, stomach, or the pillow/bed for added stability and control.

- The receiving partner sits with full penetration and rolls their hips back and forth as they straddle their partner.

- The receiving partner moves up and down, similar to the thrusting action of the penetrating partner.

- The receiving partner lies forward with their weight on the penetrating partner, and rolls their body back and forth or moves up and down. The penetrating partner (on bottom) can also place their hands on their partner's hips or butt to control the rhythm.

- The receiving partner arches backward, instead of forward, and reaches backward placing their hands on either their partner's legs or the bed for balance. The receiving partner then moves in a way that is great for stimulating the G-Spot, anus, and/or prostate.

- The receiving partner faces the opposite direction while straddling their partner, with their butt facing their partner. The receiving partner can put their hands on either the bed or their partner's legs for added balance and control.

- The receiving partner faces the opposite direction, like before, but on their hands and feet facing the ceiling (so their back is towards their partner and they are in a "spider crawl" position). They then lower their hips down enough for their partner to enter. The penetrating partner relieves some of their partner's muscular strain by supporting their hips or lower back with their hands. The penetrating partner then uses that leverage to thrust.

Powerful Non-Penetrative Positions (Wikipedia)

#1 Rubbing Together of the Genitals

Description/Variations-

- One partner positions themselves in between their partner's thighs and rubs their genitals or a similar object (such as a strap-on dildo) on their partner's genitals.
- In the case of two people with vaginas, both people face each other positioning their legs to make contact with each other's vulva in order to rub them together. Sometimes called scissoring.
- In the case of two people with penises, both people position themselves in order

to rub their penises together. Sometimes called frot or frottage.

Benefits-

- Risk of unwanted pregnancy dramatically decreases.
- Provides pleasure and intimacy for those who are uncomfortable with penetrative sexual activity.

#2 Mutual Masturbation

Description-

- Both partners lie next to each other in a way that provides easy manual stimulation of each other's genitals.
- Can lie on their backs, on their sides facing each other, both partners facing the same way, or with one partner on their back and the other on their side facing their partner.

Benefits-

- Risk of unwanted pregnancy dramatically decreases.
- Provides pleasure and intimacy for those who are uncomfortable with penetrative sexual activity.

Powerful Oral Sex Positions

#1 68-ing (variation of 69)

Description-

- Similar to the popular "69" position, where one partner lies on their back and the other straddles their genitals over their partner's face, facing the opposite direction and allowing oral access to both partner's genitals (can also be done side-by-side).
- One partner provides oral stimulation to the partner that is lying down, while they orient their body to give their partner manual access to stimulate their genitals.

Benefits-

- Good for foreplay and warming up both partners.

#2 Fellatio Variations

Description-

- The giving partner (the one performing the oral sex) lies on their back with their head hanging off the bed. The receiving partner (the one receiving the oral sex) enters their mouth while standing off the bed, allowing for thrusting. Receiving partner can also reach over and stimulate their partner's genitals at the same time. Can also be done with the giving partner lying on their stomach.

- The receiving partner (receiving oral sex) lies on their back with their legs hanging off the edge of the bed. The giving partner kneels off the bed and provides oral.

#3 Cunnilingus Variations

Description-

- The receiving partner lies on their back with a pillow (or multiple) under their butt in order to lift up their pelvis. The giving partner positions their head in between the thighs of the receiving partner.

- The receiving partner lies on their back with their legs hanging off the edge of the bed. The giving partner kneels off the bed and provides oral. The giving partner can also place the receiving partner's legs over their own shoulders.

Michael's Powerful Position

#1 Gravity

Description-

- I have never seen this position anywhere else, so as far as I'm concerned, I invented it. It's a penetrative position.

- The receiving partner is off the bed and places their shoulder blades on the ground (they are going to be practically upside down) with their back resting against the side of the bed. You may want to place a pillow underneath their head and shoulder blades.
- The receiving partner's legs are spread apart and in the air reaching towards the ceiling.
- The penetrating partner extends their legs on the bed, with their upper body hanging off the bed being supported in a horizontal manner by their hands and arms. They are now in a position to enter.
- The penetrating partner uses gravity to thrust every time they move their hips up towards the ceiling and back down.

Benefits-

- It's awesome.

Note that any of these positions can be adapted to use sex toys as well. And when attempting a new position, make sure you're taking the necessary safety precautions not to injure yourself or your partner. Some positions are acrobatic endeavors.

When you first start learning new positions, I suggest taking them one by one instead of trying to go through all of them in a single session. It can be a little stressful trying to remember ten new positions you learned that day. Focus on one at a time and you will memorize each as they become a part of your sexual arsenal.

And don't forget to have fun. Trying new positions is a great activity to share with your partner or partners. Talk about them, play around with what works and what doesn't, and find the top rotation of positions you can stick to that provide the most fun and pleasure.

Can you guess what's next?

Toys!

And no, not the Legos you used to play with. Although, I'm sure you could make something useful out of them for the bedroom.

Conclusion

If I had to pick a few main points that I think you should take away from reading this book, they would be as follows:

-Women want you to take your time and warm them up as much as possible. Do not rush sex with a woman. Quickies are fine but unless she is wet and ready the experience will not be optimal.

-Men and women both love spontaneity. Do not get into a bland routine. Try new things, especially by having sex in different and exciting places. Give your man a blowjob when he least expects it and he is sure to return the favor.

-Men are very visual, they like seeing your whole body and they love it when you are vocal during sex. Tell your man to "do you harder," to "spank you," to make you cum hard." Moan and yell your man's name and they are sure to repay you with intense sex. While giving your man head try to let him see your entire body. Suck him at an angle and let him see your bum and breasts. Do 69 with your man and allow your vagina to be directly in his face.

-Make sex a learning experience. Many couples feel that when they begin having sex, they enter a different realm. Do not allow yourself to get into this mindset. By making sex a different interaction you make it more difficult to communicate normally. Don't be afraid to laugh and joke during sex from time to time, this will lighten the mood and make it easier to vocalize exactly what you want in bed. Make time during sex to have a quick discussion on what you both want, don't want and what you might like to try.

-Watch each other masturbate. This can be an extremely helpful practice as it gives you visual information on what your partner truly likes. Sometimes it's difficult for a person to put into words how they want to be pleasured. By showing your partner what you like you leave little room for misinterpretation.

-Try anything once as long as it's not painful or potentially harmful. You should always let your partner know that he/she will not be judged for suggesting something new and taboo. Maybe you're a woman and you want to have sex with your man in front of another person, who videotapes the event, or maybe you're a man and you really want to have anal sex with your woman and you would also like her to give you a prostate massage. No matter what the suggestion is, make sure your partner knows that it's perfectly okay to suggest new sexual ideas. It's also perfectly okay to say no to ideas but I think having the rule of trying anything once (as long as it isn't painful or if it REALLY makes you uncomfortable) is a good idea. By trying anything once your partner will respect you. Let's say you try anal sex at your partner's request and you don't enjoy it. Your partner should not ask you to try it again since you have already tried and disliked it. You must respect your partner's likes and dislikes and keep an open, nonjudgmental environment in the bedroom at all times.

Sex is an important part of life and crucial for being in a fulfilling relationship. Whether you have a great sex life and just want to keep experimenting, or you're just starting to explore what makes you and your partner feel good, I hope this book has been a useful resource for you. Don't forget that this book is only a start. By opening up communication with your partner about sex, you can both continue to explore and grow sexually, figuring out how to have the most satisfying sexual relationship possible. Sex is for everyone, from flexible yogis to couch potatoes, so wink at your partner, shimmy out of your clothes, and start having fun!

Made in United States
Orlando, FL
14 January 2022